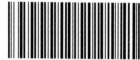

TOP 100

DRUGS IN MIDWIFERY

& WOMEN'S HEALTH

Heidi Collins Fantasia,
PhD, RN, WHNP-BC

Associate Professor
Solomont School of Nursing
University of Massachusetts, Lowell

JONES & BARTLETT
LEARNING

World Headquarters
Jones & Bartlett Learning
5 Wall Street
Burlington, MA 01803
978-443-5000
info@jblearning.com
www.jblearning.com

Jones & Bartlett Learning books and products are available through most bookstores and online booksellers. To contact Jones & Bartlett Learning directly, call 800-832-0034, fax 978-443-8000, or visit our website, www.jblearning.com.

Substantial discounts on bulk quantities of Jones & Bartlett Learning publications are available to corporations, professional associations, and other qualified organizations. For details and specific discount information, contact the special sales department at Jones & Bartlett Learning via the above contact information or send an email to specialsales@jblearning.com.

Production Credits
VP, Product Management: Amanda Martin
Director of Product Management: Matthew Kane
Product Manager: Teresa Malmberg
Product Assistant: Melina Leon
Project Manager: Jessica deMartin
Digital Products Specialist: Angela Dooley
Marketing Manager: Lindsay White
Product Fulfillment Manager: Wendy Kilborn

Composition and Project Management: S4Carlisle Publishing Services
Cover Design: Michael O'Donnell
Media Development Editor: Troy Liston
Rights & Media Specialist: John Rusk
Cover Image (Title Page): © Ilona Konstantinidi/ Shutterstock
Printing and Binding: McNaughton & Gunn
Cover Printing: McNaughton & Gunn

Library of Congress Cataloging-in-Publication Data

Names: Fantasia, Heidi Collins, author.
Title: Top 100 drugs in midwifery and women's health / Heidi Collins Fantasia.
Other titles: Top one hundred drugs in midwifery and women's health
Description: Burlington, MA : Jones & Bartlett Learning, [2021] |
Identifiers: LCCN 2019033980 | ISBN 9781284182538 (paperback)
Subjects: MESH: Pharmaceutical Preparations | Women's Health | Pregnancy | Nurses Instruction | Handbook
Classification: LCC RG528 | NLM QV 39 | DDC 618.2061--dc23
LC record available at https://lccn.loc.gov/2019033980

6048

Printed in the United States of America
23 22 21 20 19   10 9 8 7 6 5 4 3 2 1

Contents

Preface

I am grateful for the opportunity to offer this book, which is intended to provide a quick reference for some of the most common drugs utilized by women. It is my hope that both students and clinicians will find this book helpful when they are working with women. Drugs were chosen based on a variety of factors, including relevance to women's health, prevalence of underlying condition being treated, recommended use based on national guidelines, and peer-reviewed feedback. The contents are not meant to be comprehensive, and the drugs listed do not represent a personal endorsement of any medication. The full prescribing information should always be consulted as needed. Drug information changes frequently based on research and post-marketing data. Healthcare providers should always use the most current, evidence-based clinical decision making to optimize safe, women-centered care.

Drugs are listed in alphabetical order and include the indication, contraindication, mechanism of action, metabolism, excretion, adverse reactions, side effects, and major drug interactions. Also included is a section specifically related to women that discusses the use of the drug during pregnancy and lactation, as well as considerations for women who are elderly and for adolescent girls. Usual dosing and how the drug is supplied is listed. For each drug, prescribing considerations are included, which highlight important information that should be taken into account prior to use.

Relative Cost

Cost codes are provided for each drug and generally refer to a 30-day supply of a maintenance medication or short-term course of therapy. Codes are calculated using average wholesale prices (at press time in U.S. dollars) for the most common indication and route of each drug at a typical adult dosage (higher doses will be more expensive). When both generic and brand-name formulations are available, the price reflects the least expensive generic formulation. For certain products, such as the subdermal contraceptive implant and intrauterine devices, the price reflects the cost of the unit at time of purchase. ***Please use these price categories as a general guide only,*** as (1) they reflect cost, not charges; (2) pricing often varies substantially depending on location and manufacturer; and (3) private insurance, Medicaid, and Medicare coverage will vary and affect co-payment pricing and/or total cost.

Code	Cost
$	< $25
$$	$25 to $49
$$$	$50 to $99
$$$$	$100 to $199
$$$$$	> $200

Acknowledgments

I am forever grateful for the women I have worked with during the different stages of their lives. To participate in their health care is always an honor and a privilege.

I would like to thank colleagues who reviewed initial drafts and the final version of the book. Their time, attention to detail, and feedback were invaluable to the writing process.

I appreciate the support and insight of my students, colleagues, and mentors who are a great source of inspiration and encouragement. I am grateful for the unconditional love, support, and strength from my family, including my mother Gretchen Collins, my husband John, and my children Andrew, Amelia, and Evan.

Acyclovir (Zovirax)

Therapeutic class: Antiviral

Chemical class: Synthetic nucleoside analogue. Other drugs in this category include famciclovir and valacyclovir.

Indications
Acyclovir is indicated for the treatment/management of:

1. Acute herpes zoster (shingles)
2. Initial and recurrent genital herpes simplex virus (HSV)
3. Varicella (chickenpox)

Contraindications
Acyclovir is contraindicated for individuals who have a hypersensitivity to acyclovir or valacyclovir.

Mechanism of Action
In vitro, acyclovir triphosphate stops replication of herpes viral DNA. This is accomplished through inhibition of viral DNA polymerase, termination of the growing viral DNA chain, and inactivation of the viral DNA polymerase.

Metabolism & Excretion
Minimal hepatic metabolism, excreted renally mostly unchanged

Adverse Reactions
Thrombotic thrombocytopenic purpura/hemolytic uremic syndrome (TTP/HUS), which has resulted in death, has occurred for individuals who are immunocompromised and receiving acyclovir therapy.

Acute renal failure has occurred for individuals who are older, those with renal disease receiving a dose that is too high, for individuals taking other nephrotoxic drugs, and in those without adequate hydration.

Central nervous system (CNS) reactions, including agitation, confusion, delirium, hallucinations, and seizures, have been reported in individuals who are older and in those with renal disease.

Side Effects
Diarrhea, headache, nausea, and vomiting

Drug–Drug Interactions
There are no known clinically significant drug–drug interactions.

Specific Considerations for Women
Pregnancy
Acyclovir can be used during pregnancy. Based on pregnancy registry data, acyclovir does not appear to increase the rate of birth defects beyond what occurs in the general population. According to the American College of Obstetricians and Gynecologists (ACOG), women with an initial HSV outbreak or recurrent HSV during pregnancy should be offered antiviral medication to decrease the risk of perinatal transmission.

Breastfeeding
Package labeling states that acyclovir should be used with caution and only if needed by women who are breastfeeding. However, acyclovir is used for neonatal and pediatric conditions. Systemic maternal acyclovir is compatible with breastfeeding, and the amount of acyclovir excreted in human milk is only about 1% of a typical infant dose.

Adolescent women
Acyclovir can be used by adolescent women.

Elderly women
No overall differences in effectiveness for time to cessation of new lesion formation or time to healing were reported between older and younger adult individuals. The duration of pain after healing was longer for individuals over 65 years of age. Dizziness, nausea, and vomiting are reported more frequently by the elderly. Individuals who are elderly are more likely to have reduced renal function, report CNS adverse events, and require dose reductions.

Dose: Variable, based on condition being treated
Acute herpes zoster:
800 mg orally every 4 hours, 5 times daily for 7 to 10 days

A

Initial HSV outbreak:
200 mg orally every 4 hours, 5 times daily for 10 days

Episodic HSV outbreaks:
200 mg orally every 4 hours, 5 times daily for 5 days

Suppressive therapy for recurrent HSV:
400 mg orally 2 times daily for up to 12 months; doses ranging from 200 mg 3 times daily to 200 mg 5 times daily have been used as alternate therapies

Varicella:
800 mg orally 4 times daily for 5 days

How Supplied
Acyclovir is supplied as 200-mg, 400-mg, and 800-mg tablets or capsules for oral use.

Prescribing Considerations
Dose adjustments are required for individuals with decreased renal function. Acyclovir prescribing information contains dose adjustments based on creatinine clearance.

Varicella infections tend to be more severe for adolescents and adults. Initiate treatment with acyclovir within 24 hours of disease onset.

Treatment for herpes zoster (shingles) should be initiated within 72 hours of disease onset.

Genital HSV outbreaks change in frequency and severity over time. Re-evaluate the woman after 1 year of suppressive therapy to determine the need for continuation of treatment.

Episodic treatment for HSV should begin at the earliest sign (prodrome) of outbreak.

Other antiviral medication exists, such as valacyclovir, which has a less frequent dosing schedule. Choice of medication should be individualized to the specific needs of each woman.

Cost: $

Alendronate (Binosto, Fosamax, Fosamax Plus D)

Therapeutic class: Anti-osteoporotic

Chemical class: Bisphosphonate. Other medications in this category include ibandronate, risedronate, and zoledronic acid.

Indications
Alendronate is indicated for the treatment of:

1. Osteoporosis for women who are postmenopausal (also for prevention in this group)
2. Men with osteoporosis
3. Glucocorticoid-induced osteoporosis
4. Paget's disease of bone

Contraindications
Alendronate is contraindicated for women with the following conditions:

1. Abnormalities of the esophagus that delay esophageal emptying, such as achalasia or stricture
2. Inability to stand or sit upright for at least 30 minutes after taking medication
3. Increased risk of aspiration (oral solution)
4. Hypocalcemia
5. Creatinine clearance less than 35 ml/min
6. Hypersensitivity to alendronate or any component of the medication

Mechanism of Action
Alendronate binds to bone hydroxyapatite and inhibits the activity of osteoclasts, the bone-resorbing cells. Alendronate reduces bone resorption with no direct effect on bone formation. The inhibition of osteoclast activity on newly formed bone resorption surfaces reduces the number of sites where bone is remodeled. Bone formation then exceeds bone resorption at these remodeling sites, and this gradually increases bone mass.

Metabolism & Excretion
Alendronate does not undergo metabolism and is excreted renally.

Adverse Reactions
Potentially serious adverse reactions include bone, joint, and/or muscle pain; local irritation of the upper gastrointestinal (GI) mucosa, including esophageal ulcers and esophageal erosions, esophagitis, and hypocalcemia; low trauma fractures of the femoral shaft; osteonecrosis of the jaw (ONJ); and vitamin D deficiency.

Side Effects
Abdominal pain, acid reflux, diarrhea, dyspepsia, flatulence, headache, nausea, vomiting

Drug–Drug Interactions
Co-administration of alendronate and antacids, calcium supplements, or oral medications containing multivalent cations will interfere with absorption of alendronate. Women should wait at least 30 minutes after taking alendronate before taking any other oral medications.

The incidence of adverse GI events is increased with concomitant therapy of daily alendronate in doses greater than 10 mg and aspirin-containing products.

The use of nonsteroidal anti-inflammatory drugs (NSAIDs) is associated with GI irritation, and concomitant therapy with alendronate may increase the risk of adverse GI events.

Specific Considerations for Women
Pregnancy
There are no studies of alendronate that include women who are pregnant. There are no data on fetal risk in humans. However, there is a theoretical risk of fetal harm, predominantly skeletal, if a woman becomes pregnant after completing a course of bisphosphonate therapy. Women who are at risk for pregnancy should use reliable contraception.

Breastfeeding
It is not known whether alendronate is excreted in human milk, and the effects of alendronate on the infant who is breastfeeding are not known. The amount of bisphosphonate incorporated into adult bone, and therefore the amount available for release back into the systemic circulation for potential excretion into breast milk, is directly related to the dose and duration of bisphosphonate use. It is possible alendronate use may result in hypocalcemia for the infant.

Adolescent women
Alendronate is not indicated for use by adolescent women.

Elderly women
The incidence and severity of bone, joint, and muscle pain that can be associated with bisphosphonates appears to be the highest among women who are postmenopausal, but there are no recommendations for dose reductions among women over 65 years of age.

Dose: Variable, based on condition being treated
Treatment of osteoporosis for women who are postmenopausal and for men:
10 mg orally daily or 70 mg orally (tablet or 75-ml oral solution) once weekly

Prevention of osteoporosis for women who are postmenopausal:
5 mg orally daily or 35 mg orally once weekly

Glucocorticoid-induced osteoporosis:
5 mg orally daily or 10 mg orally daily for women who are postmenopausal and not receiving estrogen

Paget's disease:
40 mg orally daily for 6 months

How Supplied
Alendronate is supplied as 5-mg, 10-mg, 35-mg, 40-mg, and 70-mg tablets for oral use.
    Effervescent dissolvable tablets: 70 mg for oral use.
    Oral solution: 70 mg in 75 ml of solution for oral use.

A

Prescribing Considerations

Instructions for use will depend on the formulation prescribed, and full prescribing information should be reviewed prior to choosing alendronate. Effervescent tablets must be dissolved prior to drinking. Noneffervescent tablets are swallowed whole with a full glass of water (6 to 8 oz). No formulations should be chewed or crushed.

Effervescent tablets contain 650 mg of sodium, which is equivalent to approximately 1,650 mg sodium chloride per tablet. A different formulation (noneffervescent tablets) should be considered for women on a low-sodium or sodium-restricted diet.

Alendronate should only be taken with water. Concomitant administration of alendronate with coffee or orange juice reduces the bioavailability of alendronate by more than 50%.

Alendronate should be taken in the morning after arising. Taking the medication in the evening prior to bedtime increases the risk of esophageal erosion.

Women should wait at least 30 minutes after taking alendronate before eating, drinking, or taking other medications. Women should also remain upright for 30 minutes after taking alendronate.

Optimal duration of use has not been determined. For women who are at a lower risk for fracture, consider drug discontinuation after 3 to 5 years of use.

Discontinuing bisphosphonate treatment (including alendronate) prior to invasive dental procedures may reduce the risk for ONJ. Clinicians should consider consulting with the woman's oral surgeon to formulate a plan of care based on individual risk factors.

Women who are taking bisphosphonates (including alendronate) and present with thigh or groin pain should be evaluated for an atypical femur fracture.

The risk versus benefit of alendronate for osteoporosis prevention among individuals who are taking daily doses of glucocorticoids less than 7.5 mg of prednisone or equivalent has not been established.

Women should take supplemental calcium and vitamin D if daily dietary intake is inadequate.

Bone mineral density (BMD) assessment should be made at the initiation of therapy and repeated within 6 to 12 months for individuals who are taking a combination of alendronate and glucocorticoids. For women taking alendronate without glucocorticoids, BMD assessment should occur every 1 to 2 years during treatment.

There are many different pharmacologic treatments for osteoporosis, including other bisphosphonates. Dosing and price will vary among medications. Choice of medication should be individualized to the specific needs of each woman.

Cost: $–$$

Amitriptyline (Elavil)

Therapeutic class: Antidepressant

Chemical class: Tricyclic antidepressant (TCA). Other drugs in this category include desipramine, doxepin, imipramine, and nortriptyline.

Indications
Primary indication is for the treatment of depression.

It is used off-label for the treatment of fibromyalgia, insomnia, neuropathic pain, and vulvodynia.

Contraindications
Amitriptyline is contraindicated with a known hypersensitivity to the medication.

Amitriptyline should not be taken concomitantly with monoamine oxidase inhibitors (MAOIs).

Mechanism of Action
Amitriptyline inhibits the membrane pump mechanism responsible for uptake of norepinephrine and serotonin in adrenergic and serotonergic neurons. This may potentiate or prolong neuronal activity, and the interference

A

with reuptake of norepinephrine and/or serotonin may result in the antidepressant activity of amitriptyline.

Metabolism & Excretion
Hepatic and renal

Adverse Reactions
Potential serious adverse reactions include aggressiveness, agitation, akathisia (psychomotor restlessness), anxiety, hostility, hypomania, impulsivity, insomnia, irritability, mania, panic attacks, and worsening of depression and suicidality.

Side Effects
Most side effects are the result of anticholinergic effects, including blurred vision, constipation, drowsiness, dry mouth, exacerbation of narrow-angle glaucoma, galactorrhea, nausea, sedation, tachycardia, urinary retention, and vomiting

Drug–Drug Interactions
Hyperpyretic crises, severe convulsions, and death have occurred with individuals receiving TCAs and MAOIs simultaneously.

Amitriptyline should not be taken with cisapride due to the potential for increased QT interval and increased risk for arrhythmia.

Concomitant use of TCAs with drugs that inhibit cytochrome P450 2D6 may require lower doses than usually prescribed for either the TCA or other drug.

Cimetidine may reduce hepatic metabolism of TCAs.

Specific Considerations for Women
Pregnancy
There are no adequate, well-controlled studies of amitriptyline involving women who are pregnant, although teratogenic effects have not been seen in animal studies. Consider the use of another antidepressant agent for depression, such as sertraline, for which more safety data exist.

Breastfeeding
Amitriptyline is excreted in breast milk in low amounts. Amitriptyline use during breastfeeding is not expected to cause any adverse effects for infants who are breastfeeding, especially if the infant is older than 2 months. However, sedation is possible, especially for neonates. Other medications for depression, such as sertraline, may be considered as alternatives.

Adolescent women
Adolescent women over the age of 12 may take amitriptyline. Younger adolescents may require lower doses.

Elderly women
No differences in safety or effectiveness have been noted between older and younger women.

Individuals who are elderly are more sensitive to the anticholinergic side effects of TCAs, including amitriptyline. Cognitive impairment, confusion, delirium, psychomotor slowing, and sedation are also possible and increase the risk for falls. Therefore, individuals who are older, especially those who are over 65 years of age, should be started on low doses of amitriptyline and observed closely for adverse effects.

Dose
Initial dose for depression is usually 75 mg orally daily in divided doses. Alternately, individuals can begin treatment with 50 mg to 100 mg at bedtime. Total daily dose is 150 mg, increased gradually from the initial dose.

For younger adolescents and the elderly, lower doses are recommended, such as 10 mg orally 3 times per day and 20 mg orally at bedtime (50 mg total per day).

There are no consistent, evidence-based guidelines for off-label dosing for neuropathic pain or vulvodynia. In the literature, the most common initial dose for vulvodynia is 25 mg orally once daily, which is titrated based on the woman's response.

How Supplied
Amitriptyline is supplied as 10-mg, 25-mg, 50-mg, 75-mg, 100-mg, and 150-mg tablets for oral use.

Prescribing Considerations

Amitriptyline has a **black box warning** for an increased risk of suicidality among children, adolescents, and young adults with major depressive disorder and other psychiatric conditions.

Prior to initiating treatment with an antidepressant, individuals should be screened for bipolar disorder to reduce the risk of inducing a mixed/manic episode.

Amitriptyline should not be stopped abruptly. Gradual dose reduction over the course of 2 weeks will help prevent withdrawal symptoms of headache, malaise, and nausea.

Amitriptyline is sedating; if excessive drowsiness occurs, the medication can be taken at bedtime.

Alcohol intake should be avoided or greatly reduced while taking amitriptyline due to the risk for increased sedation.

Other TCAs are available, and dosing and price will vary among medications. Choice of medication should be individualized to the specific needs of each woman.

Cost: $$

Amoxicillin, Amoxicillin-clavulanic acid

Therapeutic class: Antibiotic

Chemical class: Penicillin; Penicillin + beta-lactamase inhibitor

Indications

Amoxicillin is indicated for the treatment of susceptible bacteria causing:

1. Infections of the ear, genitourinary tract, lower respiratory tract, nose, skin and skin structure, and throat
2. In combination for treatment of *H. pylori* infection and duodenal ulcer disease

Amoxicillin-clavulanic acid is indicated for the treatment of susceptible bacteria causing:

1. Lower respiratory tract infections
2. Acute bacterial otitis media
3. Sinusitis
4. Skin and skin structure infections
5. Urinary tract infections

Contraindications

Amoxicillin and amoxicillin-clavulanic acid are both contraindicated with a known allergy or hypersensitivity to the medication or other beta lactams (cephalosporins, penicillins).

Use of both amoxicillin and amoxicillin-clavulanic acid should be avoided by individuals with mononucleosis due to the likelihood of developing an erythematous skin rash.

Amoxicillin-clavulanic acid is contraindicated for individuals with a previous history of cholestatic jaundice or hepatic dysfunction with the medication.

Mechanism of Action

Amoxicillin is bactericidal against susceptible bacteria during the stage of active multiplication. It acts through the inhibition of cell wall biosynthesis that leads to the death of the bacteria.

Amoxicillin-clavulanic acid protects amoxicillin from degradation by some beta-lactamase enzymes and extends the antibiotic spectrum of amoxicillin to include many bacteria normally resistant to amoxicillin.

Metabolism & Excretion

Hepatic and renal

Adverse Reactions

Serious and occasionally fatal anaphylactic reactions have been reported by individuals taking penicillins.

Clostridium difficile-associated diarrhea (CDAD) has been reported with use of nearly all antibacterial agents, including amoxicillin and amoxicillin-clavulanic acid.

Hepatic dysfunction has occurred for individuals taking amoxicillin-clavulanic acid.

Side Effects
Diarrhea, nausea, rash, and vomiting. Superinfections with fungal or bacterial pathogens are possible.

Drug–Drug Interactions
Probenecid decreases the renal tubular secretion of amoxicillin, so concurrent use of both drugs may result in increased and prolonged blood levels of amoxicillin.

Amoxicillin and amoxicillin-clavulanic acid prolong prothrombin time for individuals receiving oral anticoagulation.

The concurrent administration of allopurinol and amoxicillin or amoxicillin-clavulanic acid increases the incidence of rashes for individuals receiving both drugs.

Specific Considerations for Women
Pregnancy
There is no evidence that amoxicillin or amoxicillin-clavulanic acid causes fetal harm. Both medications can be used during pregnancy.

Breastfeeding
Both amoxicillin and amoxicillin-clavulanic acid can be used during breast-feeding. Adverse reactions for the infant are rare but could include diarrhea and fungal infections.

Adolescent women
Both amoxicillin and amoxicillin-clavulanic acid are approved for pediatric use and can be taken by adolescent women.

Elderly women
No overall differences in safety or effectiveness have been observed between older and younger individuals. Both amoxicillin and amoxicillin-clavulanic acid are substantially excreted by the kidney, so the risk of adverse reactions may be increased for individuals with impaired renal function, which is more common among individuals over 65 years of age.

Dose: Variable, depending on condition being treated
Amoxicillin

Susceptible infections:
Either 250 mg or 500 mg orally every 8 hours or 875 mg orally every 12 hours.

H. pylori *infection:*
Triple therapy: 1 gram amoxicillin, 500 mg clarithromycin, and 30 mg lansoprazole, all taken orally every 12 hours for 14 days. Dual therapy: 1 gram amoxicillin and 30 mg lansoprazole, each taken orally every 8 hours for 14 days.

Amoxicillin-clavulanic acid

Susceptible infections:
Either 500 mg or 875 mg orally every 12 hours or 250 or 500 mg orally every 8 hours.

Individuals with severe renal impairment will require a dose reduction.

How Supplied
Amoxicillin is available as 250-mg, 500-mg, and 875-mg tablets or capsules for oral use.

Amoxicillin-clavulanic acid is available as 250-mg/125-mg, 500-mg/125-mg, and 875-mg/125-mg tablets for oral use.

Both amoxicillin and amoxicillin-clavulanic acid are also available as a powder for oral suspension and chewable tablets. See full product prescribing information for available doses.

Prescribing Considerations
Despite information contained in the product labeling, recent evidence **does not** support a link between non-rifampin antibiotics and hormonal contraception failure.

Adequate fluid intake will help prevent crystalluria.

Although symptoms may improve quickly with treatment, the full course of medication should be completed.

Cost: $–$$

Ampicillin

Therapeutic class: Antibiotic

Chemical class: Penicillin

Indications
Ampicillin is indicated for the treatment of susceptible bacteria causing infections of the gastrointestinal (GI), genitourinary, and respiratory tracts.

Contraindications
Ampicillin is contraindicated with a known allergy or hypersensitivity to the medication or other penicillins. It is also contraindicated for infections caused by penicillinase-producing organisms.

Mechanism of Action
Ampicillin is bactericidal against susceptible bacteria during the stage of active multiplication. It acts through the inhibition of cell wall biosynthesis that leads to the death of the bacteria.

Metabolism & Excretion
Hepatic and renal

Adverse Reactions
Serious and occasionally fatal anaphylactic reactions have been reported by individuals taking penicillins.

Clostridium difficile-associated diarrhea (CDAD) has been reported with use of nearly all antibacterial agents, including ampicillin.

Ampicillin use by individuals with mononucleosis may increase the risk of developing an erythematous skin rash.

Side Effects
Diarrhea, nausea, rash, and vomiting. Superinfections with fungal or bacterial pathogens are possible.

Drug–Drug Interactions

Probenecid decreases the renal tubular secretion of ampicillin, so concurrent use of both drugs may result in increased and prolonged blood levels of ampicillin.

The concurrent administration of allopurinol and ampicillin increases the incidence of rashes for individuals receiving both drugs.

Specific Considerations for Women

Pregnancy

There is no evidence that ampicillin causes fetal harm. It can be used during pregnancy.

Breastfeeding

Ampicillin can be used during breastfeeding. Adverse reactions for the infant are rare but could include diarrhea and fungal infections.

Adolescent women

Ampicillin is approved for pediatric use and can be taken by adolescent women.

Elderly women

No overall differences in safety or effectiveness have been observed between older and younger individuals. Ampicillin is excreted by the kidney, and the risk of adverse reactions may be increased for individuals with impaired renal function, which is more common among those over 65 years of age.

Dose

Genitourinary and GI tract infections:

The usual dose is 500 mg orally 4 times per day for 7 to 10 days.

Respiratory tract infections:

The usual dose is 250 mg orally 4 times per day for 7 to 10 days.

For infections caused by hemolytic strains of streptococci, a minimum treatment length of 10 days is recommended to decrease the risk of rheumatic fever.

Individuals with severe renal impairment will require a dose reduction.

How Supplied
Ampicillin is available in 250-mg and 500-mg capsules for oral use.

Prescribing Considerations
Despite information contained in the product labeling, recent evidence **does not** support a link between non-rifampin antibiotics and hormonal contraception failure.

Although symptoms may improve quickly with treatment, the full course of medication should be completed.

To increase absorption, ampicillin should be taken on an empty stomach.

Cost: $

Atorvastatin (Lipitor)

Therapeutic class: Antilipemic

Chemical class: HMG-CoA reductase inhibitor or statin. Other medications in this category include fluvastatin, lovastatin, pitavastatin, pravastatin, rosuvastatin, and simvastatin.

Indications
Atorvastatin is indicated to reduce:

1. The risk of angina, myocardial infarction (MI), and stroke for adults with multiple risk factors for the development of coronary heart disease (CHD)
2. The risk of MI and stroke for adults with type 2 diabetes and multiple risk factors for the development of CHD
3. The risk of nonfatal MI, fatal and nonfatal stroke, hospitalization for congestive heart failure (CHF), and angina for adults diagnosed with CHD
4. Elevated total cholesterol, low-density lipoprotein (LDL) cholesterol, apo B, and triglyceride (TG) levels and increased high-density lipoprotein (HDL) cholesterol for adults with primary hyperlipidemia (familial and nonfamilial) and mixed dyslipidemia

5. Elevated TG for adults with hypertriglyceridemia and primary dysbetalipoproteinemia
6. Total cholesterol and LDL for adults with homozygous familial hyper-cholesterolemia (HoFH)
7. Elevated total cholesterol, LDL, and apo B levels for children and adolescents 10 to 17 years of age, with heterozygous familial hyper-cholesterolemia (HeFH) when a trial of dietary changes has not been successful

Contraindications
Atorvastatin is contraindicated with:

1. Active liver disease, including unexplained persistent elevations in hepatic transaminase levels
2. Hypersensitivity to any component of this medication
3. Pregnancy and lactation

Mechanism of Action
Atorvastatin is a selective, competitive inhibitor of HMG-CoA reductase, an enzyme that converts 3-hydroxy-3-methylglutaryl-coenzyme A to mevalonate, a precursor of cholesterol. Inhibition of HMG-CoA reductase lowers the amount of mevalonate and subsequently reduces the levels of circulating total cholesterol, LDL cholesterol, and serum triglycerides.

Metabolism & Excretion
Hepatic and biliary

Adverse Reactions
Skeletal muscle effects (e.g., myopathy and rhabdomyolysis) can occur. Risks increase when higher doses are used concomitantly with cyclosporine and strong CYP3A4 inhibitors.

HMG-CoA reductase inhibitors such as atorvastatin may increase fasting serum glucose and HgbA1C levels.

Statins, such as atorvastatin, have been associated with biochemical abnormalities of liver function.

A higher incidence of hemorrhagic stroke may occur for individuals with a recent history (past 6 months) of stroke or transient ischemic attack (TIA) who are taking the highest dose of atorvastatin.

Side Effects
Diarrhea and nausea are the most commonly reported side effects.

Drug–Drug Interactions
Atorvastatin is metabolized by cytochrome P4503A4. Concomitant administration of atorvastatin and strong inhibitors of CYP3A4 (such as clarithromycin, HIV protease inhibitors, itraconazole) can increase plasma concentrations of atorvastatin.

Cyclosporine can increase the bioavailability of atorvastatin.

Atorvastatin may increase the plasma concentration of digoxin.

Gemfibrozil and colchicine may increase the risk of myopathy/rhabdomyolysis when administered with atorvastatin.

Grapefruit juice, especially in large doses, can inhibit CYP3A4 and increase plasma concentrations of atorvastatin.

Niacin may increase the risk of skeletal muscle effects. If taken with atorvastatin, a lower dose of atorvastatin should be considered.

Levels of norethindrone and ethinyl estradiol may be increased with atorvastatin. This should be considered if the woman requires contraception.

Specific Considerations for Women
Pregnancy
Atorvastatin is contraindicated for use by women who are pregnant. Safety during pregnancy has not been established and there is no apparent benefit of lipid-lowering drugs during pregnancy. HMG-CoA reductase inhibitors decrease cholesterol synthesis, and atorvastatin may cause fetal harm when administered to women who are pregnant. The medication should be discontinued as soon as pregnancy is recognized.

Breastfeeding
The consensus opinion, consistent with package labeling, is that women taking a statin should not breastfeed because of a concern with disruption of

infant lipid metabolism. However, statins have low oral bioavailability. Studies with small numbers of women have not indicated developmental issues with infants, although these data are limited. Decisions about continuing to breastfeed during statin therapy should be made on an individual basis.

Adolescent women
Atorvastatin may be used by adolescent women as indicated for the treatment of heterozygous familial hypercholesterolemia (HeFH).

Elderly women
Risks of myopathy and rhabdomyolysis increase with advanced age (over 65 years). Although no specific dose reduction is recommended for the elderly, atorvastatin should be used with caution by older adults.

Dose
The range for adults is 10 mg to 80 mg orally daily; starting dose: 10 mg or 20 mg once daily.
    The range for adolescents is 10 mg to 20 mg orally daily; starting dose: 10 mg once daily.
    Individuals requiring a large LDL reduction of more than 45% may start at 40 mg once daily.

How Supplied
Atorvastatin is supplied as 10-mg, 20-mg, 40-mg, and 80-mg tablets for oral use.

Prescribing Considerations
Risks of myopathy and rhabdomyolysis increase when higher doses are used concomitantly with cyclosporine and strong CYP3A4 inhibitors (see Adverse Reactions). To the extent possible, atorvastatin should not be used with these medications.
    Unexplained, new, and/or persistent muscle pain, tenderness, or weakness should be reported to a healthcare provider; atorvastatin should be discontinued if myopathy is diagnosed or suspected.
    Pregnancy should be avoided during treatment with atorvastatin. Reproductive-age women who could become pregnant should be counseled about the need for contraception.

Obtain liver function tests prior to beginning treatment with atorvastatin and repeat as clinically indicated during treatment. Atorvastatin should be used with caution by individuals who consume large amounts of alcohol (more than 2 alcoholic drinks/day).

Many different statins are available, and cost is variable among each medication. Choice of medication should be individualized to the specific needs of each woman.

Cost: $

Azithromycin (Zithromax, Zmax)

Therapeutic class: Antibiotic

Chemical class: Azalide macrolide

Indications
In adults, azithromycin is indicated for mild to moderate infections caused by susceptible bacteria:

1. Acute bacterial exacerbations of chronic bronchitis
2. Acute bacterial sinusitis
3. Uncomplicated skin and skin structure infections
4. Urethritis and cervicitis in adults
5. Genital ulcer disease in men
6. Community-acquired pneumonia
7. Pharyngitis/tonsillitis

Contraindications
Azithromycin is contraindicated for individuals with:

1. Hypersensitivity to azithromycin, erythromycin, any ketolide or macrolide drug
2. A history of cholestatic jaundice/hepatic dysfunction associated with prior use of azithromycin

Mechanism of Action
Azithromycin interferes with bacterial protein synthesis by binding to the 50S subunit of bacterial ribosomes.

Metabolism & Excretion
Hepatic and biliary

Adverse Reactions
Allergic reactions (some fatal), including Stevens-Johnson Syndrome (SJS) and toxic epidermal necrolysis, have been reported with azithromycin.

Prolonged cardiac repolarization and QT interval, risk of cardiac arrhythmia, and torsades de pointes have occurred with macrolide antibiotics, including azithromycin.

Clostridium difficile-associated diarrhea (CDAD) has been reported with almost all antibacterial agents, including azithromycin.

Exacerbation of symptoms of myasthenia gravis and new onset of myasthenic syndrome have been reported by individuals taking azithromycin.

Side Effects
Most common are gastrointestinal (GI) side effects of abdominal pain, diarrhea, nausea, and vomiting.

Drug–Drug Interactions
Co-administration of azithromycin and nelfinavir may increase the serum concentration of azithromycin.

Concomitant administration of azithromycin may potentiate the effects of oral anticoagulants such as warfarin. Prothrombin times should be monitored during treatment with azithromycin and oral anticoagulants.

Interactions with digoxin or phenytoin been observed with other macrolides.

Aluminum- and magnesium-containing antacids may decrease serum azithromycin concentrations.

Specific Considerations for Women
Pregnancy
Azithromycin may be used during pregnancy and animal studies have shown no increase in fetal harm.

Breastfeeding
Azithromycin is excreted in breast milk in small amounts. Azithromycin is used to treat infant and pediatric conditions and may be used while breastfeeding. It is possible that infants exposed to azithromycin via breast milk could experience diarrhea, diaper rash, and decreased appetite.

Adolescent women
Azithromycin may be used by adolescent women.

Elderly women
No differences in safety or effectiveness have been noted between older and younger women.

Individuals who are elderly may be more susceptible to development of torsades de pointes arrhythmias, but no dose adjustments are recommended for women over 65 years old.

Dose: Variable, based on condition being treated
Genital ulcer disease (chancroid):
1 gram orally in a single dose

Nongonococcal urethritis and cervicitis:
2 grams orally in a single dose

Chlamydia:
2 grams orally in a single dose

*Community-acquired pneumonia (mild), pharyngitis/tonsillitis
(second-line therapy), skin/skin structure (uncomplicated) infections:*
500 mg orally as a single dose on day 1, followed by 250 mg orally once daily on days 2 through 5

Acute bacterial exacerbations of chronic bronchitis (mild to moderate):
500 mg orally as a single dose on day 1, followed by 250 mg orally once daily on days 2 through 5 *or* 500 mg orally once daily for 3 days

Acute bacterial sinusitis:
500 mg orally once daily for 3 days

How Supplied

Azithromycin is supplied as 250-mg and 500-mg tablets for oral use.

Azithromycin oral suspension is supplied as 300-, 600-, 900-, and 1200-mg bottles. When reconstituted, the oral suspension provides either 100 mg/5 ml (300-mg bottle) or 200 mg/5 ml (600-, 900-, and 1200-mg bottles).

Prescribing Considerations

Azithromycin may be taken with or without food.

The full course of medication should be finished.

If azithromycin is prescribed to treat a sexually transmitted infection (STI), the woman's partner must be treated.

Aluminum- and magnesium-containing antacids and azithromycin should not be taken simultaneously.

GI side effects (abdominal cramping and loose, watery stools) are common.

Cost: $$

Brexanolone (Zulresso)

Therapeutic class: Antidepressant

Chemical class: Neuroactive steroid, chemically identical to allopregnanolone

Indications

Brexanolone is indicated for the treatment of moderate to severe postpartum depression (PPD).

Contraindications

There are currently no known contraindications to brexanolone other than use restricted to postpartum depression. It is not indicated for depression that occurs outside the postpartum period.

Mechanism of Action
The complete mechanism of action is unknown. Brexanolone is a modulator of GABA-A receptors. The effect of brexanolone on these receptors is thought to be the pathway for its effect on mood.

Metabolism & Excretion
Hepatic and gastrointestinal (fecal)/renal

Adverse Reactions
No postmarketing data is available for brexanolone. Therefore, information on adverse effects is limited to data from clinical trials. The most significant adverse effect was sedation and sudden loss of consciousness.

Side Effects
Dizziness, dry mouth, fatigue, headache, hot flashes/flushing, and intravenous (IV) site irritation were reported during clinical trials.

Drug–Drug Interactions
Brexanolone should not be administered with other central nervous system (CNS) depressants, including alcohol. Concomitant use with medications such as opioids, benzodiazepines, and hypnotics should be avoided. In clinical trials, use with other antidepressants increased sedation.

Specific Considerations for Women
Pregnancy
No data are available regarding brexanolone use during pregnancy but based on animal data with other drugs that enhance GABAergic inhibition, it is possible that brexanolone may cause fetal harm. A pregnancy registry has been established for women who are exposed to brexanolone during pregnancy.

Breastfeeding
Brexanolone is excreted in breast milk in low levels. Women who were breastfeeding were excluded from clinical trials. Therefore, no definitive safety data are available.

Adolescent women
The safety and efficacy of brexanolone in the treatment of PPD has not been established for adolescent women because women under the age of 18 were excluded from clinical trials.

Elderly women
Brexanolone is approved for the treatment of PPD. It is not indicated for use by women who are postmenopausal.

Dose
Administration is by continuous IV infusion over 60 hours, which is approximately 2.5 days. The dosing schedule consists of titration, maintenance, and taper in which the dose of brexanolone is gradually increased, kept steady, and then decreased during treatment.

Hours 0–4: 30 mcg/kg/hour
Hours 4–24: 60 mcg/kg/hour
Hours 24–52: 90 mcg/kg/hour or kept at 60 mcg/kg/hour for women
        who can't tolerate 90 mcg/kg/hour
Hours 52–56: 60 mcg/kg/hour
Hours 56–60: 30 mcg/kg/hour

How Supplied
Brexanolone is supplied as a solution in 100-mg/20-ml vials (5 mg/ml) for IV administration.

Prescribing Considerations
Brexanolone has a **black box warning** due to the risk for excessive sedation and sudden loss of consciousness. Because of this, brexanolone is only available through a Risk Evaluation and Mitigation Strategy (REMS) program. The requirements of this program restrict the prescription and use of brexanolone to healthcare facilities that have enrolled in the program and pharmacies that have registered with the program. Additionally, women must enroll in the program prior to infusion. Information can be found at https://www.zulressorems.com/#Public

There is a pregnancy exposure registry that monitors pregnancy outcomes for women exposed to antidepressants during pregnancy. Healthcare providers can register women by calling the National Pregnancy Registry for Antidepressants at 1-844-405-6185 or visiting online at https://womensmentalhealth.org/clinical-and-researchprograms/pregnancyregistry/antidepressants/

Specific instructions for preparation of the brexanolone infusion are provided with the medication. Brexanolone must be diluted prior to administration and infused via a dedicated IV line.

Once diluted, the product can only be stored at room temperature for 12 hours, so a 60-hour infusion will require the preparation of 5 infusion bags. A 20-ml vial (containing 100 mg of brexanolone) is placed in an infusion bag and then diluted with 40 ml of sterile water for injection and 40 ml of 0.9% sodium chloride injection. The final concentration of brexanolone in the infusion bag is 1 mg/ml. After preparation, the infusion bag can be refrigerated for 96 hours.

An infusion pump must be used to ensure accurate dosing, and continuous pulse oximetry monitoring is necessary during treatment.

Women must be supervised if they are with their infants or other children during the infusion.

Guidelines for how and when women will be transitioned to oral antidepressants postinfusion, the timing of the transition, and whether treatment with brexanolone will affect the dose of oral antidepressants have not been established.

Cost: $$$$$

Buprenorphine-naloxone (Suboxone)

Therapeutic class: Anti-addiction agent

Chemical class: Partial opioid agonist and opioid antagonist

Indications
Buprenorphine-naloxone is indicated for the treatment of opioid addiction in combination with a comprehensive treatment plan, including counseling and emotional support.

Contraindications
Buprenorphine-naloxone is contraindicated with a known allergy or hypersensitivity to either component of the medication.

Mechanism of Action
Buprenorphine is a partial opioid agonist, and naloxone is an opioid antagonist.

Metabolism & Excretion
Hepatic and renal

Adverse Reactions
Neonatal abstinence syndrome (NAS) can occur for infants exposed to buprenorphine-naloxone prenatally.

Opioid withdrawal symptoms will occur with abrupt discontinuation of buprenorphine-naloxone.

Other possible adverse effects include adrenal insufficiency, elevation of cerebrospinal spinal fluid (CSF), hepatitis, orthostatic hypotension, and overdose for opioid-naïve individuals.

Side Effects
Constipation, edema, glossodynia, insomnia, oral hypoesthesia, oral mucosal edema, pain, withdrawal symptoms

Drug–Drug Interactions
Buprenorphine-naloxone should not be used in combination with other central nervous system (CNS) depressants such as alcohol, benzodiazepines, and opioids.

Concomitant use of buprenorphine-naloxone and serotonergic drugs may result in serotonin syndrome.

Concomitant use of buprenorphine-naloxone and CYP3A4 inhibitors can increase the plasma concentrations of buprenorphine. Conversely, concomitant use of buprenorphine-naloxone and CYP3A4 inducers can decrease the plasma concentrations of buprenorphine.

Non–nucleoside reverse transcriptase inhibitors (NNRTIs) are metabolized by CYP3A4. Concomitant use of NNRTIs and buprenorphine-naloxone may require close monitoring of the buprenorphine-naloxone dose.

The use of monoamine oxidase inhibitors (MAOIs) and buprenorphine-naloxone may increase the risk of serotonin syndrome.

Specific Considerations for Women

Pregnancy

Women who are pregnant can use buprenorphine-naloxone as part of medication-assisted treatment (MAT) for opioid addiction. Women should be advised of the risk of NAS among infants exposed to buprenorphine-naloxone prenatally. Untreated opioid addiction during pregnancy is associated with preterm birth, low birth weight infants, and fetal death. The risk of NAS should be weighed against known adverse outcomes of untreated opioid addiction.

Breastfeeding

Buprenorphine is present in low levels in breast milk and naloxone is poorly absorbed. Generally, women who are stable on MAT and adherent to treatment are encouraged to breastfeed if able to. The infant should be monitored for sedation.

Adolescent women

The safety and efficacy of buprenorphine-naloxone has not been established for women under age 18.

Elderly women

No differences in response to treatment have been noted between older and younger individuals. Individuals who are older may be more susceptible to sedation and adverse effects due to decreases in hepatic and renal function that occur with aging.

Dose

Day 1: An induction dosage of buprenorphine-naloxone up to 8 mg/2 mg is recommended. Consider starting with doses of 2 mg/0.5 mg or 4 mg/1 mg and titrate up every 2 hours under direct supervision until the buprenorphine-naloxone dose up to 8 mg/2 mg dose is reached.

Day 2: A single daily dose of buprenorphine-naloxone up to 16 mg/4 mg is recommended.

Day 3 and onward: Progressive adjustments in the dose of buprenorphine-naloxone in amounts of 2 mg/0.5 mg or 4 mg/1 mg can be made to suppress opioid withdrawal symptoms.

The recommended target dose during maintenance treatment is buprenorphine-naloxone 16 mg/4 mg.

The sublingual route should be used during medication induction to minimize the exposure to the naloxone component, which can precipitate withdrawal symptoms.

How Supplied

Buprenorphine-naloxone is available in sublingual film for sublingual or buccal use in the following strengths:

buprenorphine 2 mg/naloxone 0.5 mg
buprenorphine 4 mg/naloxone 1 mg
buprenorphine 8 mg/naloxone 2 mg
buprenorphine 12 mg/naloxone 3 mg

Prescribing Considerations

Buprenorphine-naloxone is a Schedule III controlled substance.

Under the Drug Addiction Treatment Act (DATA) of 2000, prescription of buprenorphine-naloxone for the treatment of opioid dependence is limited to healthcare providers who meet qualifying requirements, including the completion of buprenorphine waiver training.

Healthcare providers who prescribe buprenorphine-naloxone should limit refills, especially during initial treatment, to reduce the risk of abuse. Consider follow-up visits in the office at least weekly during initial treatment.

The first dose of buprenorphine-naloxone sublingual film should be administered when objective signs of moderate opioid withdrawal appear, but not less than 6 hours after the individual has taken the last dose of opioids.

When determining the prescription quantity for unsupervised treatment at home, consider the individual's risk of misuse, stability in treatment, security of home environment, likelihood of diversion, the ability to safely and correctly manage a supply of buprenorphine-naloxone, and frequency of follow-up visits.

Buprenorphine-naloxone must be allowed to dissolve completely and shouldn't be chewed, cut, or swallowed whole.

If there are children in the home where buprenorphine-naloxone sublingual film will be stored, caution must be taken to ensure that children do not inadvertently ingest the film, which could result in a fatal overdose.

Buprenorphine-naloxone may impair mental and physical abilities. Individuals should avoid activities that require mental alertness until it is known how they will react to buprenorphine-naloxone.

Cost: $$$$–$$$$$

Bupropion (Wellbutrin, Zyban)

Therapeutic class: Antidepressant and antismoking agent

Chemical class: Aminoketone

Indications
Bupropion is indicated for the treatment of major depressive disorder (MDD) and smoking cessation.

Contraindications
Bupropion is contraindicated for individuals with a seizure disorder; a current or prior history of bulimia or anorexia nervosa; concurrent abrupt withdrawal of alcohol, benzodiazepines, barbiturates, or antiepileptic drugs; concurrent or past 14-day use of monoamine oxidase inhibitors (MAOIs); and those with known hypersensitivity to bupropion or any component of the medication.

Mechanism of Action
Bupropion is a relatively weak inhibitor of the neuronal reuptake of norepinephrine and dopamine. The exact mechanism by which bupropion assists with smoking cessation and depression is presumed to be related to noradrenergic and/or dopaminergic mechanisms.

Metabolism & Excretion
Hepatic and renal

Adverse Reactions
Significant adverse reactions are possible. Neuropsychiatric symptoms of agitation, depression, hallucinations, hostility, mania, psychosis, and suicidal ideation have occurred. Individuals with a history of mental health disorders may experience increased adverse reactions.

Seizures can occur with bupropion treatment.

Angle-closure glaucoma, hypersensitivity reactions, and hypertension have occurred.

Side Effects
Dry mouth, insomnia, skin rashes

Drug–Drug Interactions
Bupropion is primarily metabolized by CYP2B6. Bupropion may interact with drugs that are inhibitors or inducers of CYP2B6.

Clopidogrel and ticlopidine may increase bupropion levels. Carbamazepine, efavirenz, lopinavir, phenobarbital, phenytoin, and ritonavir may decrease bupropion levels.

Other drug interactions exist. Full prescribing information should be consulted.

Specific Considerations for Women
Pregnancy
Data from epidemiological studies that included women who were exposed to bupropion in the first trimester of pregnancy indicate no increased risk of congenital malformations overall. Untreated depression and smoking during pregnancy both carry risks to the fetus. Need for the medication should be evaluated and weighed with known risks of maternal depression and smoking during pregnancy.

Breastfeeding
Bupropion is excreted in small amounts in breast milk and is not expected to cause adverse effects for the infant. Women taking bupropion may breastfeed, but infants should be monitored for jitteriness, sedation, and vomiting.

Adolescent women

Bupropion may be used by adolescent women. Adolescents should be monitored closely for mood changes and suicidality.

Elderly women

No dose adjustments are recommended for women over age 65. No differences in safety or effectiveness have been noted between older and younger women.

Dose: Variable, depending on condition being treated

Smoking cessation:

Bupropion should be initiated one week prior to chosen quit date. Usual starting dose is 150 mg orally once daily for 3 days. Dose can be increased to 150 mg twice daily (every 12 hours).

MDD:

Usual starting dose is 100 mg orally twice daily. After 3 days, the dose may be increased to 100 mg 3 times per day (with at least 6 hours between each dose). Usual target dose is 300 mg daily in divided doses.

Maximum dose for smoking cessation is 300 mg orally daily, in 3 divided doses of 100 mg. Maximum dose for MDD is 450 mg orally daily, in 3 divided doses of 150 mg.

Moderate to severe hepatic impairment: 75 mg orally once daily for MMD or 150 mg orally every other day for smoking cessation.

How Supplied

Bupropion is available as 75-mg and 100-mg tablets for oral use.

Prescribing Considerations

Bupropion has a **black box warning** for risk of suicidal thoughts and behaviors for children, adolescents, and young adults. Monitor for worsening mood disorders and suicidal thoughts.

Bupropion is marketed under two different brand names, Zyban for smoking cessation and Wellbutrin for depression. Each indication has different doses and prescribers should be cautious when selecting the correct dose and treatment length.

Prior to initiating treatment with bupropion, individuals should be screened for bipolar disorder, to reduce the risk of inducing a mixed/manic episode.

When used for smoking cessation, women should be evaluated after an initial 12 weeks of treatment. If they have been successful in complete tobacco cessation, treatment is advised for an additional 12 weeks to increase the likelihood of long-term smoking cessation.

If women are unable to completely quit smoking with treatment, smoking should gradually be reduced over the course of 12 weeks.

Bupropion may be used with a nicotine replacement system.

Tablets should not be chewed or crushed.

Smokers who relapse after quitting may repeat treatment with bupropion.

Women with mild hepatic or renal impairment may require a reduced dose.

Cost: $$

Carboprost tromethamine (Hemabate)

Therapeutic class: Oxytocic

Chemical class: Prostaglandin

Indications

Carboprost is indicated for aborting pregnancy between the 13th and 20th weeks of gestation in the following conditions related to second-trimester abortion:

1. Failure of expulsion of the fetus during treatment with another method
2. Premature rupture of membranes in intrauterine methods with loss of drug and insufficient or absent uterine activity
3. Requirement of a repeat intrauterine instillation of drug for expulsion of the fetus
4. Inadvertent or spontaneous rupture of membranes in the presence of a previable fetus and absence of adequate activity for expulsion

Carboprost is also indicated for the treatment of postpartum hemorrhage due to uterine atony that has not responded to conventional methods of management, including intravenous (IV) oxytocin, uterine massage, and ergot medications.

Contraindications
Carboprost is contraindicated for women with known hypersensitivity to the product, in the presence of acute pelvic inflammatory disease (PID), and for women with active cardiac, pulmonary, renal, or hepatic disease.

Carboprost is not feticidal. It is not indicated for termination of pregnancy once the infant has reached viability.

Mechanism of Action
Carboprost stimulates myometrial contractions. For termination of pregnancy, these contractions assist in evacuation of the products of conception from the uterus. For postpartum hemorrhage, the myometrial contractions provide hemostasis at the site of placental attachment.

Metabolism & Excretion
Hepatic and renal

Adverse Reactions
When carboprost is used for the termination of pregnancy, the abortion may be incomplete in approximately 20% of cases.

In the setting of chorioamnionitis, carboprost may be less effective in controlling postpartum hemorrhage.

Uterine rupture has occurred in rare cases.

Side Effects
Diarrhea and vomiting are common, reported by up to 60% of women treated with carboprost.

Other side effects may include abdominal pain/cramping, bronchospasm, chills, dizziness, flushing, hypersensitivity reactions, syncope, and vaginal bleeding. Transient pyrexia and elevation in blood pressure may occur.

Drug–Drug Interactions
Concomitant use with other oxytocic agents is not recommended.

Specific Considerations for Women

Pregnancy
Carboprost does not appear to be teratogenic, but the uterotonic effects will stimulate uterine contractions. It should only be administered to women who are pregnant in the setting of pregnancy termination.

Breastfeeding
It is not known if carboprost is excreted into breast milk. There is no information available to guide decisions regarding use for postpartum hemorrhage and breastfeeding. However, blood levels peak quickly after administration of carboprost and decline within 2 hours after a single dose.

Adolescent women
Carboprost has not been studied for women under age 18.

Elderly women
Women who are postmenopausal are not pregnant and therefore carboprost provides no therapeutic benefit.

Dose

Abortion of previable fetus:
One ampule (250 mcg) of carboprost in a deep intramuscular (IM) injection is given as an initial dose. Subsequent doses of 250 mcg should be given at intervals of 1.5 and 3.5 hours based upon uterine response. The total dose and length of treatment should not exceed 12 mg over the course of 2 days.

Postpartum hemorrhage:
One ampule (250 mcg) of carboprost in a deep IM injection. Repeated doses may be given based on clinical outcomes but should not exceed 2 mg (8 doses).

How Supplied

Carboprost is supplied as a sterile solution in 1-ml ampules (250 mcg) for IM use.

Prescribing Considerations

Carboprost has a **black box warning** for adherence to recommended dosages that are used by trained healthcare providers in a hospital or other setting where immediate intensive care and surgical facilities are present.

In addition to stimulating uterine smooth muscle, carboprost also stimulates the smooth muscle of the GI tract. This most likely produces the vomiting and/or diarrhea that are common side effects. Pretreatment or concurrent administration of antiemetic and antidiarrheal drugs decreases the very high incidence of GI effects that occur with carboprost. Use of antiemetic and antidiarrheal drugs should be considered an integral part of the treatment plan for women who are administered carboprost.

The uterine cramping that results from carboprost may be significant enough to require medication, such as nonsteroidal anti-inflammatory drugs (NSAIDs) or acetaminophen, to decrease discomfort.

Cost: $$$–$$$$

Ceftriaxone for injection (Rocephin)

Therapeutic class: Antibiotic

Chemical class: Cephalosporin

Indications
Ceftriaxone is indicated for a variety of infections caused by susceptible organisms:

1. Uncomplicated gonorrhea
2. Pelvic inflammatory disease
3. Lower respiratory tract infections
4. Acute bacterial otitis media
5. Skin infections
6. Urinary tract infections
7. Bacterial septicemia
8. Bone and joint infections
9. Intra-abdominal infections
10. Meningitis

Contraindications

Ceftriaxone is contraindicated for individuals with a known allergy to cephalosporins. It should be used with caution by individuals with a known hypersensitivity to penicillin and those with a history of gastrointestinal disease, especially colitis.

Mechanism of Action

Ceftriaxone is bactericidal and inhibits bacterial cell wall synthesis.

Metabolism & Excretion

Negligible metabolism; renal and biliary excretion

Adverse Reactions

Clostridium difficile-associated diarrhea (CDAD) has been reported with antibacterial agents, including ceftriaxone, and may be life-threatening. Bloody diarrhea, colitis, and diarrhea may occur.

Sonographic abnormalities of the gallbladder and pancreatitis/biliary obstruction have been reported.

An immune-mediated hemolytic anemia has been observed when individuals receive cephalosporin-class antibacterials, including ceftriaxone.

Side Effects

With intramuscular (IM) administration, burning, induration, pain, and redness may occur at the injection site. Other side effects include diarrhea, thrush, vaginal candidiasis infection, and vulvovaginitis.

Drug–Drug Interactions

If administering ceftriaxone intravenously (IV), the medication cannot be given simultaneously with calcium-containing solutions.

The concomitant use of warfarin with many classes of antibiotics, including cephalosporins, may increase the international normalized ratio (INR) and potentiate the risk for bleeding.

Ceftriaxone may increase cyclosporin levels.

Specific Considerations for Women

Pregnancy

Ceftriaxone can be used during pregnancy.

Breastfeeding
Ceftriaxone has been detected in human breast milk in low levels. Women can breastfeed during treatment, but ceftriaxone has the potential to alter the infant's gastrointestinal flora. Infants who are breastfeeding should be monitored for bloody stools, candidiasis, and diarrhea.

Adolescent women
Ceftriaxone can be used by adolescent women.

Elderly women
No differences in safety or effectiveness have been noted between older and younger women.

Dose: Variable; depends on condition being treated.
Uncomplicated gonococcal infections:
A single IM dose of 250 mg

Pelvic inflammatory disease:
A single IM dose of 250 mg as part of an outpatient treatment protocol with other antibiotics.

Other infections:
For adults, the usual daily dose is 1 to 2 grams given IM once a day (or in divided doses twice a day) depending on the type and severity of infection. The total daily dose should not exceed 4 grams.

How Supplied
Ceftriaxone is supplied as a powder in glass vials as 250-mg, 500-mg, 1-gram, or 2-gram equivalents of ceftriaxone. When reconstituted for IM injection, each 1 ml of solution contains either 250 mg/ml or 350 mg/ml of ceftriaxone depending on the amount of diluent added.

Prescribing Considerations
For IM administration, ceftriaxone should be injected deep into a large muscle; aspiration will help avoid unintentional injection into a blood vessel.

Common diluents for IM use include sterile water for injection and 1% lidocaine solution without epinephrine.

Once reconstituted, the solution should be used within 24 hours.

Although potentially inconvenient, women will need to return to the office for the IM injection when ceftriaxone is used as part of an outpatient treatment regimen for PID or gonorrhea.

Cost: $–$$

Cetirizine (Zyrtec and many generic brands)

Therapeutic class: Antihistamine

Chemical class: Second-generation histamine H1 antagonist. Other medications in this class include fexofenadine and loratadine.

Indications
Cetirizine is indicated for the relief of nasal and non-nasal symptoms associated with seasonal or perennial allergic rhinitis for adults and children.

Cetirizine is also used for the treatment of urticaria.

Contraindications
Cetirizine is contraindicated for individuals with a known allergy or hypersensitivity to the medication.

Mechanism of Action
The principal effects of cetirizine are mediated via selective inhibition of H1 receptors with minimal anticholinergic and antiserotonergic activity.

Metabolism & Excretion
Hepatic and renal

Adverse Reactions
No serious or life-threatening adverse reactions have been noted.

Side Effects
Dizziness, drowsiness, dry mouth, fatigue, and somnolence are possible.

Drug–Drug Interactions
Use with other central nervous system (CNS) depressants, such as alcohol, could potentiate drowsiness.

Specific Considerations for Women
Pregnancy
Animal models do not suggest that cetirizine is teratogenic during pregnancy. Cetirizine is generally considered acceptable during pregnancy if first-generation antihistamines are not tolerated.

Breastfeeding
Small, occasional doses of cetirizine are acceptable during breastfeeding. Larger doses for a prolonged time may cause drowsiness for the infant or decreased milk supply.

Adolescent women
Cetirizine is approved for use by children and appropriate for adolescent women.

Elderly women
No differences in safety or effectiveness have been noted between older and younger women. However, half-life may be prolonged for the elderly, probably related to decreased renal function.

Dose
A usual dose for allergic rhinitis and idiopathic urticaria is 10 mg orally daily.
    Cetirizine may be taken daily or on an as-needed basis, depending on the severity of allergy symptoms.

How Supplied
Cetirizine is available over the counter as 10-mg tablets for oral use. Liquid formulations for children are also available.

Prescribing Considerations
Although second-generation antihistamines are usually considered to be nonsedating, some individuals will report dizziness or drowsiness after taking cetirizine.

Anticholinergic effects are less than with first-generation antihistamines, but women may experience vaginal dryness.

Other over-the-counter second-generation antihistamines exist with similar dosing schedules. Choice of medication should be individualized to the specific needs of each woman.

Cost: $

Ciprofloxacin (Cipro, Cipro XR)

Therapeutic class: Antibiotic

Chemical class: Fluoroquinolone

Indications
Ciprofloxacin has *in vitro* activity against a wide range of gram-negative and gram-positive microorganisms. It is used to treat a variety of conditions, including infections of the abdomen, bones, joints, lower respiratory tract, prostate, sinuses, skin, and urinary tract. Ciprofloxacin is used for the treatment of gonorrhea, infectious diarrhea, and typhoid fever. Additionally, ciprofloxacin is used for postexposure treatment for inhalation anthrax.

Ciprofloxacin XR is indicated only for the treatment of urinary tract infections, including acute uncomplicated pyelonephritis.

Contraindications
Ciprofloxacin is contraindicated for individuals with a history of hypersensitivity to ciprofloxacin, any quinolone, or any component of the medication.

Concomitant administration with tizanidine is contraindicated.

Mechanism of Action
The bactericidal action of ciprofloxacin results from inhibition of the enzymes topoisomerase II and topoisomerase IV, which are required for bacterial DNA replication, transcription, repair, and recombination.

Metabolism & Excretion
Hepatic and renal

Adverse Reactions
Serious and fatal hypersensitivity (anaphylactic) reactions have been reported by individuals taking quinolones, including ciprofloxacin.

Central nervous system (CNS) events such as confusion, convulsions, depression, dizziness, hallucinations, increased intracranial pressure, psychosis, suicidal thoughts or acts, and tremors have been reported by individuals receiving quinolones, including ciprofloxacin.

Clostridium difficile-associated diarrhea (CDAD) has been reported with use of nearly all antibacterial agents, including ciprofloxacin.

Generalized weakness, paresthesias, peripheral neuropathy, tendonitis, and tendon rupture have been reported with ciprofloxacin.

Side Effects
Ciprofloxacin may cause moderate to severe photosensitivity/phototoxicity reactions, including exaggerated sunburn reactions involving areas exposed to light. Other side effects include diarrhea, nausea, rash, and vomiting.

Overgrowth of fungi can occur and result in oral thrush and vulvovaginal candidiasis.

Drug–Drug Interactions
Concurrent administration of antacids containing magnesium hydroxide or aluminum hydroxide may reduce the bioavailability of ciprofloxacin by as much as 90%.

Concomitant administration of ciprofloxacin with theophylline decreases the clearance of theophylline, resulting in elevated serum theophylline levels. Serious and fatal reactions have occurred. Concomitant use of ciprofloxacin and theophylline should be avoided if possible. If the two medications must be given concurrently, serum theophylline levels should be monitored, and dosage adjustments made, as appropriate.

Co-administration of ciprofloxacin and other drugs primarily metabolized by CYP1A2, such as methylxanthines and tizanidine, results in increased plasma concentrations of the co-administered drug.

Specific Considerations for Women
Pregnancy
There are no adequate, well-controlled studies of ciprofloxacin use by women who are pregnant. Therapeutic doses during pregnancy are unlikely to pose a substantial teratogenic risk. Other antibiotics with more safety data should be used first. However, ciprofloxacin may be considered if it is the only acceptable choice.

Breastfeeding
Use of ciprofloxacin is acceptable for women who are breastfeeding. Infants should be monitored for possible effects on the gastrointestinal flora, such as candidiasis (diaper rash, thrush) or diarrhea. Avoiding breastfeeding for 3 to 4 hours after a dose will further decrease the infant's exposure to ciprofloxacin in breast milk.

Adolescent women
Ciprofloxacin is approved for pediatric use and thus can be used by adolescent women.

Elderly women
Individuals over age 60 may be at a higher risk of tendonitis and spontaneous tendon rupture, especially if they are also taking corticosteroids.

Dose: Variable, depends on condition being treated
In general, doses range from 250 mg to 750 mg orally every 12 hours. Duration of treatment typically ranges from 7 to 14 days, depending on the infection being treated. If the XR formulation is used, ciprofloxacin is taken every 24 hours.

For postexposure treatment of inhalation anthrax, 500 mg is given orally every 12 hours for 60 days.

See full prescribing information for doses and length of treatment pertaining to individual infections and for dose adjustments for individuals with renal impairment.

How Supplied
Ciprofloxacin is supplied as 250-mg, 500-mg, and 750-mg tablets for oral use.

Ciprofloxacin XR is supplied as 500-mg and 1,000-mg tablets for oral use.

Ciprofloxacin is also available in an oral suspension and solution for intravenous (IV) infusion.

Prescribing Considerations

Ciprofloxacin has a **black box warning** for an increased risk of tendonitis and tendon rupture among individuals of all age groups. The risk is increased for individuals over age 60; those taking corticosteroids; and recipients of heart, lung, and kidney transplants.

Individuals taking ciprofloxacin should be well hydrated to prevent the formation of highly concentrated urine and crystalluria.

Individuals should avoid exposure to sunlight or artificial ultraviolet light to reduce the risk of photosensitivity reactions.

The full course of medication should be completed even if symptoms resolve.

Ciprofloxacin should not be taken with dairy products or calcium-fortified juices, as absorption of ciprofloxacin may be significantly reduced. Antacids containing magnesium hydroxide or aluminum hydroxide will also decrease the absorption of ciprofloxacin.

Cost: $–$$

Clindamycin hydrochloride (Cleocin)
Clindamycin vaginal cream (Cleocin Vaginal Cream 2%)
Clindamycin vaginal ovules (Cleocin Vaginal Ovules)

Therapeutic class: Antibiotic

Chemical class: Semisynthetic lincosamide

Indications

Clindamycin hydrochloride is indicated for the treatment of serious infections caused by susceptible strains of pneumococci, staphylococci, and streptococci. These include pelvic, respiratory, skin, and soft tissue infections.

Clindamycin vaginal cream/ovules are indicated for the treatment of bacterial vaginosis (BV).

Contraindications
Clindamycin oral capsules and vaginal cream/ovules are contraindicated for women with a history of hypersensitivity to clindamycin, lincomycin, or any of the components of the cream/ovule. These formulations are also contraindicated for individuals with a history of regional enteritis, ulcerative colitis, or a history of colitis associated with antibiotic use.

Mechanism of Action
Clindamycin is predominantly bacteriostatic and inhibits bacterial protein synthesis.

Metabolism & Excretion
Hepatic and renal

Adverse Reactions
Hypersensitivity reactions can include anaphylaxis, skin rashes, and urticaria.

Pseudomembranous colitis has been reported with antibacterial agents, including clindamycin, and may be life-threatening. Bloody diarrhea, colitis, and diarrhea have occurred with the use of all forms (oral, parenteral, topical, vaginal) of clindamycin. A toxin produced by *Clostridium difficile* is a primary cause of colitis associated with antibiotic use.

Side Effects
Oral thrush, vaginal candidiasis infection, and vulvovaginitis can occur with use of all formulations. Local burning, edema, and itching can occur with use of vaginal clindamycin.

Drug–Drug Interactions
Systemic clindamycin has been shown to have neuromuscular blocking properties. The vaginal preparations should be used with caution by women receiving other neuromuscular blocking medications.

Specific Considerations for Women

Pregnancy

Oral clindamycin can be used by women who are pregnant if indicated and no other antibiotics are appropriate. Although data are conflicting, the use of vaginal clindamycin preparations by women who are pregnant is often restricted to the second and third trimesters. According to the CDC STD Treatment Guidelines, metronidazole is the first-line medication for the treatment of symptomatic BV during pregnancy.

Breastfeeding

Clindamycin has been detected in human breast milk after oral and parenteral administration. It is not known if clindamycin is excreted in breast milk following the use of the vaginal cream/ovules. Women can breastfeed during treatment, but clindamycin has the potential to alter the infant's gastrointestinal flora. Infants who are breastfeeding should be monitored for bloody stools, candidiasis, and diarrhea.

Adolescent women

Clindamycin oral and vaginal preparations can be used by adolescent women.

Elderly women

Individuals who are older may be more susceptible to treatment-related diarrhea with oral clindamycin and should be monitored closely. There have been no reported treatment-related differences between women who are younger and older who are using clindamycin vaginal cream/ovules.

Dose

The recommended dose of the vaginal cream is one applicatorful of clindamycin vaginal cream (approximately 100 mg of clindamycin phosphate) intravaginally, preferably at bedtime, for 3 or 7 consecutive days by women who are not pregnant and for 7 consecutive days by women who are pregnant.

The recommended dose of the vaginal ovules is one ovule (100 mg clindamycin) intravaginally, preferably at bedtime, for 3 consecutive days.

The recommended dose of oral clindamycin for serious infections is 150 mg to 300 mg orally every 6 hours. For severe infections, the dose can be increased to 450 mg orally every 6 hours. Treatment length is determined by the specific infection being treated and ranges from 7 to 10 days.

How Supplied

Clindamycin vaginal cream is supplied as a 40-gram tube with 7 disposable applicators.

Clindamycin vaginal ovules are supplied as a box of 3 suppositories and one applicator.

Clindamycin capsules are supplied in doses of 75 mg, 150 mg, or 300 mg.

Prescribing Considerations

Oral preparations:

Clindamycin hydrochloride for oral use has a **black box warning** due to the association with severe colitis and the development of *Clostridium difficile*-associated diarrhea. It should be reserved for severe infections in which no other antibacterial agent is appropriate.

Vaginal preparations:

Approximately 5% of the clindamycin dose is systemically absorbed from the vagina. Consider a diagnosis of pseudomembranous colitis for women who develop diarrhea after treatment with vaginal clindamycin cream/ovules.

Vaginal intercourse should be avoided during treatment with clindamycin vaginal cream/ovules.

Clindamycin vaginal cream/ovules may be used during menses, but tampons will absorb the medication and should be avoided.

Clindamycin vaginal cream/ovules contain mineral oil that may weaken latex condoms or diaphragms. Use of latex condoms and diaphragms should be avoided during treatment with clindamycin vaginal cream/ovules and for 72 hours after treatment has been completed.

Cost: $–$$

Clobetasol propionate (Temovate and many others)

Therapeutic class: Topical anti-inflammatory

Chemical class: Corticosteroid

Indications
Clobetasol is a super-high-potency topical steroid used for:

1. The relief of inflammatory and pruritic manifestations of corticosteroid-responsive dermatoses for individuals over 12 years of age
2. Treatment of moderate to severe plaque-type psoriasis for individuals over 16 years of age

Contraindications
Use with caution on broken or atrophied skin.

Mechanism of Action
Topical corticosteroids exhibit anti-inflammatory, antipruritic, and vasoconstrictive properties. Topical corticosteroids reverse vascular dilation and permeability and inhibit collagen deposition and keloid formation. These actions result in decreased edema, erythema, plaque formation and scaling of the affected skin, and pruritus.

Metabolism & Excretion
Hepatic and renal

Adverse Reactions
Due to its high potency, clobetasol has been associated with suppression of the hypothalamic-pituitary-adrenal axis (HPA).

Systemic absorption can increase the risk for Cushing's syndrome, glucosuria, and hyperglycemia.

Side Effects
Local skin reactions may include acne, burning/stinging, contact dermatitis, erythema, folliculitis, hypertrichosis, hypopigmentation, miliaria, perioral dermatitis, secondary infections, skin fissures, and striae dermatitis.

Drug–Drug Interactions
There are no major drug-drug interactions. However, clobetasol shouldn't be combined with other corticosteroids.

Specific Considerations for Women
Pregnancy
Topical corticosteroids, including clobetasol, should not be used in large amounts, on large areas, or for prolonged periods of time during pregnancy. Mild- to moderate-potency agents are recommended over super-high-potency corticosteroids and should be used for short durations.

Breastfeeding
Extensive and prolonged application of potent corticosteroids may cause systemic effects for the woman, but it is unlikely that short-term application of topical corticosteroids poses a risk to an infant who is breastfeeding through excretion into breast milk. It is advisable to use the least potent drug on the smallest area of skin possible and ensure that the infant's skin does not come into direct contact with the areas of skin that have been treated. Consider the use of a lower potency topical steroid (hydrocortisone) if possible and appropriate.

Adolescent women
Adolescent women may use clobetasol if other modalities to treat plaque psoriasis have failed.

Elderly women
No dose adjustments are recommended based on age. However, the skin of individuals who are older may be atrophied and more susceptible to adverse skin reactions associated with high-potency topical corticosteroids. The lowest effective dose for the shortest time is prudent.

Dose
Inflammatory and pruritic manifestations:
A thin layer is applied to the affected skin twice daily (morning and night) for up to 2 weeks.

Moderate to severe plaque psoriasis:
A thin layer is applied to the affected skin twice daily (morning and night) for up to 4 weeks.

Vulvar lichen sclerosus:
Clobetasol cream: A thin layer is applied to the affected labial, perineal, and vulvar areas twice daily, once in the morning and once at night. Treatment is limited to 2 consecutive weeks. Amounts greater than 50 grams per week should not be used. Intermittent clobetasol applications may be needed to maintain results.

Clobetasol ointment: A thin layer is applied to the vulvar areas for 3 months in the following pattern: once daily for the first month, then on alternate days for the second month, and then twice weekly for the third month. An alternate effective regimen is clobetasol applied once daily for 3 months; if symptoms resolve in less than 3 months, the ointment can be applied twice weekly for the remainder of the treatment period.

For all conditions, amounts greater than 50 grams per week should not be used.

How Supplied
Clobetasol cream is supplied in strengths of 0.025% and 0.05% in 30- and 60-gram tubes.

Clobetasol ointment is supplied in a 0.05% strength in 15- and 30-gram tubes.

Prescribing Considerations
Clobetasol should not be combined with other corticosteroids.

HPA suppression is more common with high doses used on large body areas.

Clobetasol is not appropriate for the treatment of acne or rosacea.

The lowest dose for the shortest time should be used. Intermittent evaluation of treatment response is prudent.

Cost: $$–$$$

Clomiphene citrate (Clomid, Serophene)

Therapeutic class: Ovulatory stimulant

Chemical class: Chlorotrianisene derivative

Indications
Clomiphene is indicated with demonstrated ovulatory dysfunction for women desiring pregnancy who meet the following criteria:

1. Not pregnant
2. No ovarian cysts (women with ovarian enlargement due to polycystic ovary syndrome [PCOS] may use clomiphene)
3. No abnormal vaginal bleeding
4. Normal liver function

Contraindications
Clomiphene citrate is contraindicated with a known allergy or hypersensitivity to the drug or its components.

Additional contraindications include abnormal vaginal bleeding of undetermined origin, liver disease or a history of liver dysfunction, ovarian cysts or enlargement not resulting from PCOS, the presence of a pituitary tumor, or uncontrolled thyroid or adrenal dysfunction.

Mechanism of Action
Clomiphene initiates a series of endocrine events that cause a preovulatory gonadotropin surge and subsequent follicular rupture. These events include an increase in the release of pituitary gonadotropins, growth of the ovarian follicle, and an increase in the circulating level of estradiol. Estrogenic and antiestrogenic properties of clomiphene probably have a role in the initiation of ovulation.

Metabolism & Excretion
Hepatic and renal

Adverse Reactions
Ovarian hyperstimulation syndrome (OHSS) has been reported with clomiphene. This potentially fatal condition can progress quickly, and women should be monitored for early warning signs, which include abdominal pain and distention, diarrhea, nausea, and vomiting.

Clomiphene may increase the risk of ovarian cysts and can enlarge uterine fibroids. Multifetal pregnancy is possible.

Side Effects
Abdominal pain, breast discomfort, nausea, vasomotor flushing, and visual changes.

Drug–Drug Interactions
There are no known clinically significant drug–drug interactions.

Specific Considerations for Women
Pregnancy
Clomiphene is contraindicated during pregnancy because once pregnancy is established, the drug provides no therapeutic benefit. Available data do not suggest an increased risk of birth defects for fetuses inadvertently exposed to clomiphene.

Breastfeeding
Clomiphene appears to lower serum prolactin. It is likely that clomiphene would interfere with lactation for a woman who is breastfeeding. Women who are breastfeeding should not take clomiphene.

Adolescent women
There are no specific guidelines for adolescents with PCOS and ovulatory dysfunction who wish to become pregnant. Lifestyle changes, including weight loss, should be considered a first-line treatment.

Elderly women
Clomiphene is not indicated for women who are postmenopausal. Women who are perimenopausal and have declining estrogen levels will have a decreased response to clomiphene.

Dose
The usual starting dose is 50 mg orally once daily for 5 days, beginning on day 5 of the menstrual cycle. The dose should be increased only if ovulation is not achieved with the 50-mg dose. Maximum dose is 100 mg orally daily for 5 days.

Women with PCOS may have an exaggerated response to clomiphene and should be started on the lowest recommended dose and treated for the shortest duration.

How Supplied
Clomiphene is supplied as 50-mg tablets for oral use.

Prescribing Considerations
Clomiphene is most effective for women with PCOS and amenorrhea associated with galactorrhea, psychogenic factors, and cases of secondary amenorrhea of undetermined etiology.

Prior to prescribing clomiphene, other causes of infertility or subfertility should be investigated.

Irregular menses are common with ovulatory dysfunction. Other reasons for the abnormal bleeding, such as cervical or endometrial neoplasia, should be ruled out.

A pelvic examination, in conjunction with sonography, may help establish and/or monitor ovarian enlargement.

Women with lower estrogen levels, such as women who are perimenopausal, may respond less favorably to clomiphene.

Ovulation most often occurs 5 to 10 days after a course of clomiphene. Intercourse should be timed to coincide with the expected ovulation.

If ovulation does not occur after three courses of clomiphene, treatment should be discontinued. Total length of treatment should not exceed 6 cycles.

Cost: $$

Copper intrauterine device (Paraguard T 380A)

Therapeutic class: Contraceptive

Chemical class: Metal

Indications
The copper intrauterine device (IUD) is indicated for long-term contraception, for up to 10 to 12 years of use.

Contraindications
The copper IUD should not be used with:

1. Pregnancy or suspected pregnancy
2. Abnormalities of the uterus resulting in distortion of the uterine cavity
3. Acute pelvic inflammatory disease (PID), or current behavior suggesting a high risk for PID
4. Postpartum endometritis or postabortal endometritis in the past 3 months
5. Known or suspected uterine or cervical malignancy
6. Vaginal bleeding of unknown etiology
7. Mucopurulent cervicitis
8. Wilson's disease
9. Allergy to any component of the IUD
10. A previously placed IUD that has not been removed

Mechanism of Action
Copper is continuously released into the uterine cavity. Mechanisms by which copper enhances contraceptive efficacy include interference with sperm transport and fertilization of an egg, and possibly prevention of implantation.

Metabolism & Excretion
Renal (minimal excretion of copper)

Adverse Reactions

Although the risk of pregnancy is low, if a pregnancy does occur with the copper IUD there is a greater risk of it being ectopic.

PID and sepsis are possible. Embedment, expulsion, and perforation have occurred.

Side Effects

The copper IUD will alter the menstrual bleeding pattern. Heavier menses and dysmenorrhea are most common, especially during the first year of use.

Other possible side effects include abdominal pain and cramping, anemia, backache, vaginal discharge, and vasovagal reactions with insertion.

Drug–Drug Interactions

There are no known clinically significant drug–drug interactions.

Specific Considerations for Women

Pregnancy

The copper IUD is contraindicated during pregnancy. If a pregnancy is diagnosed with an IUD in place, the IUD should be removed to decrease the chance of sepsis. IUD removal may lead to pregnancy loss.

Breastfeeding

The copper IUD can be used by women who are breastfeeding.

Adolescent women

Adolescent women can use the copper IUD.

Elderly women

Women who are postmenopausal do not require contraception, and the copper IUD provides no therapeutic benefit.

Dose

Each copper IUD has a total exposed copper surface area of 380 ± 23 mm^2. It is approved for 10 years of use but evidence-based for 12 years.

How Supplied

The copper IUD is supplied as a single unit.

Prescribing Considerations

The technique for inserting the copper IUD differs from those used for other types of available IUDs. Providers should receive specific training on the IUD they are inserting.

Nucleic acid amplification testing (NAAT) for gonorrhea and chlamydia should be obtained at insertion if women have not had routine screening or if they have risk factors for STIs based on their history. Infections should be treated appropriately, but insertion should not be delayed while waiting for test results. The greatest risk for PID is within the first 21 days after insertion if there is an active cervical infection.

The copper IUD can be placed at any time during the menstrual cycle if the provider is reasonably certain the woman is not pregnant. Documenting a negative pregnancy test prior to insertion is prudent. The IUD can also be placed immediately after birth or surgical abortion. The copper IUD can be placed as soon as medical abortion is confirmed.

The copper IUD can be used for emergency contraception if placed within 5 days of unprotected intercourse.

Consider offering a follow-up appointment approximately 6 weeks after insertion to assess any concerns. Although this visit is not medically necessary, it does allow for a discussion of any bothersome side effects, including changes in the menstrual cycle. However, women can decide individually if they are interested in a postinsertion visit.

Heavy menstrual bleeding that does not lessen after one year may not improve. Consider removing the IUD in the presence of significant anemia or prolonged, heavy bleeding.

The IUD should be removed or changed after the appropriate time (10 to 12 years).

Review possible adverse reactions, including expected changes in bleeding pattern.

The copper IUD does not protect against sexually transmitted infections (STIs) or HIV.

Cost: $$$$$

Denosumab (Prolia)

Therapeutic class: Immunological agent

Chemical class: Human IgG2 monoclonal antibody; osteoclast inhibitor (RANKL [receptor activator of nuclear factor kappa-B ligand] inhibitor)

Indications

For women, denosumab is approved to treat:

1. Postmenopausal osteoporosis with high risk for fracture
2. Bone loss while receiving adjuvant aromatase inhibitor therapy for breast cancer
3. Glucocorticoid-induced osteoporosis while taking systemic glucocorticoids in a daily dosage equivalent to 7.5 mg or greater of prednisone for at least 6 months.

Contraindications

Denosumab is contraindicated for women who are pregnant, have hypocalcemia, or have a systemic hypersensitivity to any component of the product.

Mechanism of Action

Denosumab binds to RANKL, a soluble protein essential for the formation, function, and survival of osteoclasts, the cells responsible for bone resorption. Denosumab prevents RANKL from activating its receptor, RANK, on the surface of osteoclasts and their precursors. Prevention of the RANKL/RANK interaction inhibits osteoclast formation and function and decreases bone resorption. This increases bone mass and strength in cortical and trabecular bone.

Metabolism & Excretion

Minimal

Adverse Reactions

Serious adverse reactions have occurred. These include:

1. Hypersensitivity and anaphylaxis
2. Hypocalcemia and mineral abnormalities (phosphorus and magnesium)

3. Osteonecrosis of the jaw
4. Atypical, low-trauma femoral fractures
5. Vertebral fractures following discontinuation of treatment
6. Serious infections leading to hospitalization
7. Dermatologic reactions, including dermatitis, eczema, rash, and urticaria
8. Musculoskeletal pain, which could be severe and disabling
9. Suppression of bone remodeling

D

Side Effects
Fatigue, muscle and back pain, weakness

Drug–Drug Interactions
Denosumab is also marketed under the name Xgeva, which has a different dose and indication. Both medications should not be taken together.

Other calcium-lowering medications should not be used with denosumab.

Specific Considerations for Women
Pregnancy
There are no well-controlled studies of denosumab that included women who are pregnant. Based on animal data, denosumab may cause fetal harm and is contraindicated during pregnancy. Women who are premenopausal should use effective contraception during treatment and for 5 months after the last injection.

Breastfeeding
There is no information about the presence of denosumab in human milk. Due to the lack of information regarding effects on milk production and infants who are breastfeeding, evaluation of all available options for the prevention and treatment of osteoporosis should be considered for women who are breastfeeding.

Adolescent women
Denosumab is not indicated for use by adolescent women.

Elderly women
No differences in safety or effectiveness have been noted between older and younger women.

Dose
A 60-mg dose of denosumab is injected subcutaneously (SQ) by a health-care provider in the woman's upper arm, upper thigh, or abdomen every 6 months.

How Supplied
Supplied as a single-use, prefilled syringe containing 60 mg of denosumab in a 1-ml solution.

Prescribing Considerations
Women should take a calcium supplement of 1,000 mg and at least 400 international units (IU) of vitamin D daily during treatment with denosumab. Preexisting hypocalcemia must be corrected prior to beginning treatment with denosumab.

Serum calcium, phosphorus, and magnesium levels should be monitored during treatment if women are at risk for alterations in mineral metabolism (thyroid or parathyroid surgery, hyperparathyroidism, malabsorption syndromes, significant renal impairment).

Denosumab should not be used by women who are pregnant. A negative pregnancy test should be documented prior to treatment if the woman is premenopausal and pregnancy is possible.

Although osteonecrosis of the jaw can occur spontaneously, it is generally associated with dental procedures such as tooth extractions, dental surgery, and dental implants. Preventative dentistry is encouraged prior to treatment. Women should be encouraged to maintain good oral hygiene and regular, preventative dentistry.

Denosumab is marketed under two brand names: Prolia for prevention of osteoporosis and Xgeva for skeletal events related to certain malignancies. Prescribers need to be cautious when choosing the correct dose and indication.

Women should be advised to report any new onset of groin, hip, or thigh pain during treatment.

Cost: $$$$$

Depot medroxyprogesterone acetate injection (Depo Provera)

Therapeutic class: Contraceptive

Chemical class: Progestin

Indications
Depot medroxyprogesterone acetate (DMPA) is indicated for the prevention of pregnancy. The subcutaneous (SQ) formulation is also indicated for the management of endometriosis-related pain.

Contraindications
DMPA is contraindicated with:

1. Known or suspected pregnancy
2. Undiagnosed vaginal bleeding
3. Known or suspected malignancy of breast
4. Active thrombophlebitis, current/past history of thromboembolic disorders, or cerebral vascular disease
5. Significant liver disease
6. Known hypersensitivity to medroxyprogesterone acetate or any of its other ingredients.

Mechanism of Action
DMPA inhibits the secretion of gonadotropins. This prevents follicular maturation and ovulation and results in endometrial thinning.

Metabolism & Excretion
Hepatic

Adverse Reactions
There are many potential adverse reactions that should be considered:

1. DMPA reduces serum estrogen levels and is associated with decreased bone mineral density (BMD). A **black box warning** has been issued for this effect.

2. Although DMPA is a progestin-only method of contraception, there have been severe thrombotic events associated with use.
3. Ectopic pregnancy.
4. Menstrual irregularities, including amenorrhea, irregular and unpredictable bleeding, and spotting.
5. Weight gain.
6. Decrease in glucose tolerance.
7. Depression.
8. Delayed ovulation and return to fertility after discontinuation.
9. Anaphylaxis.

Side Effects
Abdominal pain, acne, bloating, breast tenderness, fatigue, hair loss, headache, and pain at injection site have been reported.

Drug–Drug Interactions
Co-administration of HIV protease inhibitors and non-nucleoside reverse transcriptase inhibitors (NNRTIs) may cause either an increase or decrease in plasma levels of progestins.

Aminoglutethimide may decrease serum levels of DMPA.

Other drugs that induce CYP3A4 enzymes may decrease the effectiveness of hormonal contraceptives. These include barbiturates, bosentan, carbamazepine, felbamate, griseofulvin, oxcarbazepine, phenytoin, rifampin, St. John's wort, and topiramate.

Specific Considerations for Women
Pregnancy
DMPA is a contraceptive and therefore not indicated during pregnancy. However, if a woman is inadvertently exposed to DMPA during early pregnancy, there appears to be little or no increased risk of birth defects in the fetus above the rate that occurs in the general population.

Breastfeeding
Progestin-only contraceptives, such as DMPA, are considered the hormonal method of choice during lactation if a woman does not want to use a

nonhormonal method. DMPA does not adversely affect the quality or quantity of breast milk. Product labeling states that DMPA should not be initiated prior to 6 weeks postpartum, but U.S. Medical Eligibility Criteria for Contraceptive Use lists DMPA as either a category 2 (less than 1 month postpartum) or category 1 (more than 1 month postpartum) recommendation.

Adolescent women

DMPA may be used by adolescent women. Safety and efficacy have been established for women after menarche. Adolescence is a critical period of bone accretion. It is unknown if use of DMPA by adolescent women will reduce peak bone mass and increase the risk of osteoporotic fractures in later life. U.S. Medical Eligibility Criteria for Contraceptive Use lists DMPA as a category 2 recommendation for women under age 18. Length of treatment should be determined individually.

Elderly women

DMPA is indicated for contraception and therefore is not appropriate for women who are postmenopausal and not at risk for pregnancy.

Dose

105 mg intramuscularly (IM) every 3 months (13 weeks)
or
104 mg SQ every 3 months (12 to 14 weeks)

How Supplied

DMPA for IM use is supplied in 1-ml vials or prefilled syringes containing 150 mg DMPA.

DMPA for SQ use is supplied as a prefilled syringe containing 104 mg of DMPA.

Prescribing Considerations

DMPA has a **black box warning** for loss of BMD. This loss may not be completely reversible after extended use. It is unknown if loss of BMD increases the risk for osteoporotic fracture later in life. Package labeling recommends that use be limited to no more than 2 years due to the decrease in

BMD. However, if no other contraceptive method is appropriate, use may be extended.

Women should be assessed for osteoporosis risk factors, including tobacco and alcohol use, eating disorders, metabolic disease, family history, and medications associated with bone loss. It is unknown if supplemental calcium and vitamin D decrease DMPA-associated bone loss or prevent future fractures.

The IM formulation should be injected deep into either the deltoid or gluteal muscle.

The SQ formulation should be injected at a 45-degree angle into either the abdomen or upper thigh.

Progestins can interfere with laboratory testing, and DMPA therapy should be noted when specimens are submitted.

Women should be counseled about potential adverse effects and how to manage them.

Women who are considering a pregnancy soon should understand that DMPA has been associated with a longer return to fertility compared with other contraceptive methods. A short-acting reversible method may be more appropriate for women considering pregnancy in the next 12 months.

DMPA does not protect against sexually transmitted infections (STIs).

Cost: $$–$$$

Doxycycline (Doryx, Oracea, Monodox, Vibramycin, and others)

Therapeutic class: Antibiotic

Chemical class: Tetracycline

Indications
Doxycycline is indicated for the treatment of a variety of infections, including rickettsial, sexually transmitted infections (STIs), respiratory tract, and ophthalmic infections. It is also indicated for inhalational anthrax (post-exposure); as adjunctive treatment with acute intestinal amebiasis, severe

acne, prophylaxis of malaria; as an alternative treatment for selected infections when penicillin is contraindicated; and in other susceptible bacterial infections.

Contraindications
Doxycycline is contraindicated for individuals with hypersensitivity to any tetracycline.

Mechanism of Action
Tetracyclines, including doxycycline, are primarily bacteriostatic and probably exert an antimicrobial effect by the inhibition of protein synthesis. Doxycycline is effective against a wide range of gram-positive and gram-negative organisms.

Adverse Reactions
Clostridium difficile-associated diarrhea (CDAD) and pseudomembranous colitis have been reported with antibacterial agents, including doxycycline. Antibiotics alter the normal flora of the colon, leading to overgrowth of *C. difficile*.

Anemia, benign intracranial hypertension, hypersensitivity, skin reactions, and transient increases in blood urea nitrogen (BUN) have been reported.

Side Effects
Gastrointestinal (GI) reactions are common, including anorexia, diarrhea, dysphagia, glossitis, nausea, and vomiting.

Overgrowth of nonsusceptible organisms, including fungi, is possible. This can result in anogenital monilial infections, oral thrush, and vulvovaginal candidiasis.

Photosensitivity and exaggerated sunburn reactions have been reported with the use of tetracyclines.

Drug–Drug Interactions
Doxycycline may reduce the effectiveness of penicillin.

Tetracyclines may depress plasma prothrombin activity when taken with anticoagulants.

Barbiturates, carbamazepine, and phenytoin may decrease the half-life of doxycycline.

Antacids containing aluminum, bismuth subsalicylate, calcium, iron-containing preparations, and magnesium interfere with the absorption of doxycycline.

Concurrent use of doxycycline and methoxyflurane may cause fatal renal toxicity.

Specific Considerations for Women

Pregnancy
Tetracycline drugs, including doxycycline, should not be used during fetal, infant, and childhood tooth development because they can cause permanent discoloration of teeth. Therefore, doxycycline should not be taken during pregnancy except in the case of anthrax infection or exposure if no other drugs are acceptable.

Breastfeeding
Short-term use of doxycycline by women who are breastfeeding is acceptable. Short-term use is not likely to be harmful because drug levels are low and absorption by the infant is inhibited by the calcium in breast milk. Prolonged or repeat courses during lactation should probably be avoided. Infants who are breastfeeding should be monitored for rash and for possible effects on the gastrointestinal flora, such as candidiasis or diarrhea (diaper rash, thrush).

Adolescent women
Adolescent women may use doxycycline. It can be used after age 8.

Elderly women
No differences in safety or effectiveness have been noted between older and younger women. In general, dose selection for an individual who is older should start at the low end of the dosing range.

Dose: Variable, depending on condition being treated

Chlamydia:
100 mg orally twice daily for 7 days

Syphilis:
Individuals who are penicillin-allergic, unable to be desensitized, and have early syphilis should be treated with doxycycline 100 mg orally twice daily for 2 weeks. Individuals with syphilis of one or more years duration should be treated with doxycycline 100 mg orally twice daily for 4 weeks. Penicillin remains the first-line choice.

Inhalation anthrax:
100 mg orally twice daily for 60 days

Other infections:
The usual dose is 100 mg orally twice daily (every 12 hours) on the first day of treatment, followed by 100 mg orally daily for the remainder of treatment.

Severe infections may require doses of 100 mg orally every 12 hours for the entire course of treatment.

How Supplied
Doxycycline is available in 20-mg, 40-mg, 50-mg, 60-mg, 75-mg, 100-mg, 150-mg, and 200-mg tablets and capsules for oral use.

Prescribing Considerations
Despite information contained in the product labeling, recent evidence **does not** support a link between nonrifampin antibiotics and hormonal contraception failure.

If taken for an STI, sexual activity should be avoided until treatment has been completed by all partners.

Individuals should avoid natural sunlight and artificial ultraviolet light to avoid the risk of excessive sunburn.

GI upset is common. Doxycycline may be taken with food.

The entire course of medication must be completed, even if symptoms resolve.

Symptoms of CDAD should be reported to a healthcare provider.

Cost: $–$$

Doxylamine/pyridoxine hydrochloride (Diclegis)

Therapeutic class: Antiemetic

Chemical class: Doxylamine succinate is classified as an antihistamine and pyridoxine hydrochloride is a vitamin B6 analogue.

Indications
Doxylamine succinate/pyridoxine hydrochloride is indicated for the treatment of nausea and vomiting of pregnancy (NVP) that is unresponsive to conservative management, including dietary and lifestyle modifications.

Contraindications
Doxylamine succinate/pyridoxine is contraindicated for women with a known sensitivity to any of the ingredients or ethanolamine-derivative antihistamines. Doxylamine succinate/pyridoxine should not be used with monoamine oxidase inhibitors (MAOIs).

Doxylamine succinate/pyridoxine has anticholinergic properties and should be used with caution by women with asthma, increased intraocular pressure, narrow-angle glaucoma, pyloroduodenal obstruction, stenosing peptic ulcer, and urinary bladder-neck obstruction.

Mechanism of Action
The exact mechanism of action of doxylamine succinate/pyridoxine hydrochloride is not known. The vomiting center in the medulla of the brain receives signals through multiple neurotransmitters, including histamine. When the pathway of the neurotransmitters is interrupted, the vomiting reflex is decreased or eliminated. As an antihistamine, doxylamine may interrupt the histamine pathway and reduce vomiting. How vitamin B6 reduces nausea is unclear.

Metabolism & Excretion
Hepatic and renal

Adverse Reactions
No serious adverse reactions have been reported.

Side Effects
The most common side effects are dizziness, severe drowsiness, and somnolence.

Drug–Drug Interactions
MAOIs prolong and intensify the anticholinergic (drying) effects of anti-histamines. Central nervous system (CNS) depressants such as alcohol, hypnotics, opioids, other antihistamines, and sedatives will potentiate drowsiness and should be avoided.

Specific Considerations for Women
Pregnancy
Doxylamine succinate/pyridoxine is indicated for use during pregnancy and there is no evidence that it causes fetal harm.

Breastfeeding
Doxylamine succinate/pyridoxine passes into breast milk, and irritability or sedation of infants who are breastfeeding is possible. Decisions about using doxylamine succinate/pyridoxine to control NVP while breastfeeding should be made on an individual basis and consider the severity of maternal symptoms, age of the infant, and frequency of breastfeeding.

Adolescent women
The safety and effectiveness of doxylamine succinate/pyridoxine has not been established for women under age 18. Use by adolescents who are pregnant should be made on an individual basis and consider all options to control NVP.

Elderly women
Doxylamine succinate/pyridoxine is indicated for the treatment of NVP and therefore not appropriate for women who are postmenopausal.

Dose
Day 1: Two tablets orally at bedtime
Day 2: Two tablets orally at bedtime
Day 3: One tablet orally in the morning and 2 tablets orally at bedtime (if symptoms not controlled with previous dose)

Day 4: One tablet orally in the morning, one tablet orally in mid-afternoon, and 2 tablets orally at bedtime (if symptoms not controlled with previous dose)

The maximum daily dose is 4 tablets (1 morning, 1 mid-afternoon, 2 at bedtime).

How Supplied
The delayed-release tablets are supplied as a single strength of 10 mg doxylamine succinate and 10 mg pyridoxine hydrochloride for oral use.

Prescribing Considerations
Doxylamine succinate/pyridoxine is meant to be taken as a daily medication and not on an as-needed basis.

Significant drowsiness and somnolence are possible, especially if a woman is taking doxylamine succinate/pyridoxine during the daytime. Women should be cautioned to avoid activities that require mental alertness until they know how the medication will affect them.

Taking doxylamine succinate/pyridoxine with food delays absorption. When possible, this medication should be taken on an empty stomach. Because of the delayed-release action, doxylamine succinate/pyridoxine should not be crushed or cut.

Use of doxylamine succinate/pyridoxine may cause a false positive immunoassay drug screen result for methadone, opiates, and phencyclidine ([PCP], angel dust). Confirmatory testing should be performed if a woman is taking doxylamine succinate/pyridoxine and drug screening is done during pregnancy.

Cost: $$$$$

Dulaglutide (Trulicity)

Therapeutic class: Antidiabetic

Chemical class: Glucagon-like peptide 1 (GLP-1) agonist. Other drugs in this category include liraglutide and semaglutide.

Indications
Dulaglutide is indicated for the improvement of glycemic control and the prevention of major cardiovascular events for adults with type II diabetes.

Contraindications
Dulaglutide is contraindicated for individuals with a personal or family history of medullary thyroid carcinoma or multiple endocrine neoplasia syndrome type 2.

Dulaglutide should not be used for the treatment of type I diabetes and is not a substitute for insulin.

Dulaglutide should not be used by individuals with a serious hypersensitivity reaction to the medication or its components.

Mechanism of Action
Dulaglutide activates the GLP-1 receptor in pancreatic beta cells. Dulaglutide increases intracellular cyclic AMP (cAMP) in beta cells, leading to glucose-dependent insulin release; decreases glucagon secretion; and slows gastric emptying.

Metabolism & Excretion
Hepatic and renal

Adverse Reactions
Serious adverse reactions are possible and include acute cholecystitis, acute pancreatitis, acute renal failure, hypoglycemia (especially when used with sulfonylureas or insulin), and thyroid C-cell tumors.

Side Effects
Gastrointestinal (GI) reactions are common and include abdominal pain, bloating, constipation, diarrhea, dyspepsia, flatulence, nausea, and vomiting. Dulaglutide slows gastric emptying and has not been studied for individuals with gastroparesis.

Other side effects can include dizziness, fatigue, headache, and injection-site discomfort and redness.

Drug–Drug Interactions
Dulaglutide causes delayed gastric emptying and therefore has the potential to affect the absorption of concomitantly administered oral medications.

Specific Considerations for Women

Pregnancy

There is limited information on the use of dulaglutide for glucose control during pregnancy and, based on animal studies, the potential for fetal harm exists. Other antidiabetic medications should be considered if glucose control is needed during pregnancy. The American College of Obstetricians and Gynecologists (ACOG) and the American Diabetes Association (ADA) continue to recommend human insulin as the standard of care for women diagnosed with gestational diabetes mellitus (GDM) who require treatment beyond dietary and lifestyle modifications.

Breastfeeding

It is not known if dulaglutide is excreted into human milk. Dulaglutide is a large peptide molecule and therefore the amount in breast milk is likely to be very low. Additionally, absorption is unlikely because any ingested drug is probably destroyed in the infant's gastrointestinal tract. If glucose control is necessary during lactation, other oral antidiabetic medications or insulin should be considered.

Adolescent women

The safety and efficacy of dulaglutide have not been established for individuals under age 18.

Elderly women

No differences in safety or effectiveness have been noted between older and younger women.

Dose

The recommended starting dose of dulaglutide is 0.75 mg once weekly, injected subcutaneously (SQ) into the abdomen, thigh, or upper arm. The maximum dose is 1.5 mg once weekly.

How Supplied

Dulaglutide is supplied as prefilled, single-dose pens for SQ injection. Pens are available in doses of 0.75 mg/0.5 ml and 1.5 mg/0.5 ml.

Prescribing Considerations
Dulaglutide has a **black box warning** for risk of thyroid C-cell tumors in mice. Dulaglutide should not be prescribed for individuals with a personal or family history of medullary thyroid cancer or for individuals with multiple endocrine neoplasia syndrome type 2.

Dulaglutide should not be used as a first-line pharmacologic treatment for glucose control if interventions beyond dietary and lifestyle changes are warranted.

Dulaglutide pens should be stored in the refrigerator.

A missed dose of dulaglutide should be given as soon as possible if there are at least 72 hours before the next dose is scheduled. If less than 3 days remain prior to the next dose, the missed dose should be skipped and given on the regularly scheduled day.

Other GLP-1 agonists are available for the treatment of type II diabetes. Decisions about which medication is appropriate should be made individually with women and consider cost, dosing schedule, and individual preference.

Cost: $$$$$

Elagolix (Orilissa)

Therapeutic class: Analgesic

Chemical class: Gonadotropin releasing hormone (GnRH) receptor antagonist

Indications
Elagolix is indicated for the management of moderate to severe pain associated with endometriosis.

Contraindications
Elagolix is contraindicated for women with osteoporosis, severe hepatic impairment, and women who are pregnant. It should not be used with strong organic anion transporting polypeptide (OATP) 1B1 inhibitors.

Mechanism of Action
Elagolix binds to GnRH receptors in the pituitary gland. The blockage of GnRH signaling suppresses the production of luteinizing hormone (LH) and follicle-stimulating hormone (FSH), which then decreases estradiol and progesterone. The partial to full dose-dependent estrogen suppression that results from elagolix helps to control dysmenorrhea and pelvic pain associated with endometriosis.

Metabolism & Excretion
Hepatic and renal

Adverse Reactions
A decrease in bone mineral density (BMD) occurs while taking elagolix, and elevations in alanine aminotransferase (ALT) may also occur. Suicidal ideation, suicidal thoughts, and worsening of mood disorders are possible.

Side Effects
Elagolix will cause a change in menstrual bleeding and can result in lighter or irregular menses. Vasomotor symptoms may occur due to a reduction in estrogen levels.

Drug–Drug Interactions
Elagolix is a weak to moderate inducer of cytochrome P450 (CYP) 3A and a substrate of certain cytochromes and protein transporters. Co-administration with elagolix may decrease plasma concentrations of drugs that are substrates of CYP3A.

Elagolix may increase digoxin levels and decrease levels of midazolam and rosuvastatin.

Rifampin may increase levels of elagolix, and concomitant use of the 200-mg dose is not recommended. Elagolix 150 mg daily may be used with rifampin for a maximum of 6 months.

Estrogen-containing contraception reduces the efficacy of elagolix.

Specific Considerations for Women
Pregnancy
Exposure to elagolix early in pregnancy may increase the risk of early pregnancy loss, and the medication should not be used during pregnancy. If a

woman is interested in taking elagolix, treatment should begin within the first 7 days of the menstrual period to preclude the possibility of pregnancy. If a woman is beyond the first week of her menstrual cycle, a pregnancy test should be done prior to treatment.

Breastfeeding
It is not known if elagolix is present in breast milk or if there are any effects on the infant who is breastfeeding. Women who are breastfeeding and are seeking treatment for endometriosis-related pain should speak with their healthcare provider about available options.

Adolescent women
The safety and efficacy of elagolix have not been established for adolescents under age 18.

Elderly women
Women who are postmenopausal do not have a menstrual cycle and endometriosis regresses. Elagolix is not appropriate for women who are postmenopausal.

Dose
Recommended dosing is based on liver function.

Normal liver function or mild hepatic impairment:
150 mg orally once daily for up to 24 months or 200 mg orally twice daily for up to 6 months

Moderate hepatic impairment:
150 mg orally once daily for up to 6 months

How Supplied
Elagolix is available in 150-mg and 200-mg tablets for oral use.

Prescribing Considerations
Treatment with elagolix should begin within the first seven days of a woman's menstrual period to preclude the possibility of pregnancy. If a woman is beyond the first week of her menstrual cycle, a pregnancy test should be

done prior to treatment and elagolix started if the healthcare provider is reasonably certain the woman is not pregnant.

Contraception is required while taking elagolix. The hypoestrogenic effects of elagolix may result in early pregnancy loss, so women who are considering a pregnancy should not begin treatment.

Estrogen-containing contraception (patch, pills, or ring) may decrease the effectiveness of elagolix and should not be used while taking the medication and for one week after the completion of treatment. Contraceptive methods not containing estrogen should be advised during treatment.

Ovulation may be suppressed for women taking elagolix, but this is not consistent, and women should not rely on elagolix for contraception.

Mild vasomotor symptoms may result from lower estrogen levels. Personal and environmental modifications in clothing and temperature will help manage symptoms.

Irregular and lighter menses are common, and monitoring menstrual cycles for fertility awareness may be difficult.

A missed dose should be taken as soon as remembered, but doses should not be doubled.

Decreased BMD occurs during treatment with elagolix. It is not known if this increases a woman's overall risk of fracture or whether supplementation with calcium and vitamin D is advisable or necessary.

Cost: $$$$$

Emtricitabine and tenofovir disoproxil fumarate (Truvada)

Therapeutic class: Antiretroviral

Chemical class: Nucleoside analog reverse transcriptase inhibitors

Indications
Emtricitabine-tenofovir (FTC/TDF) is indicated in the following situations:

1. In combination with other antiretroviral agents for the treatment of HIV-1 infection for adults and children weighing at least 17 kg (37 lb).

2. In combination with safer sex practices for HIV-1 pre-exposure prophylaxis (PrEP) to reduce the risk of sexually acquired HIV-1 for at-risk adults and adolescents weighing at least 35 kg (77 lb).

Contraindications

FTC/TDF is contraindicated for PrEP for individuals with unknown or HIV-positive status.

FTC/TDF for HIV-1 PrEP is not recommended for individuals with estimated creatinine clearance less than 60 ml/min.

FTC/TDF is not recommended for individuals who are HIV-positive with estimated creatinine clearance below 30 ml/min or for individuals who are HIV-positive and requiring hemodialysis.

Mechanism of Action

Emtricitabine inhibits viral reverse transcriptase and is active in vitro on HIV-1. Tenofovir disoproxil fumarate inhibits viral reverse transcriptase and acts as a DNA chain terminator.

Metabolism & Excretion

Hepatic and renal

Adverse Reactions

Tenofovir disoproxil fumarate, one component of FTC/TDF, has been associated with Fanconi syndrome, renal failure, and renal impairment.

Tenofovir disoproxil fumarate has been associated with a decrease in bone mineral density (BMD) and an increase in biochemical markers of bone metabolism and greater bone turnover. Cases of osteomalacia associated with proximal renal tubulopathy have been reported.

Severe acute exacerbations of hepatitis B (HBV), including liver decompensation and liver failure, have been reported by individuals infected with HBV who have discontinued FTC/TDF.

Individuals treated for HIV-1 infection with combination antiretroviral medication, including FTC/TDF, have developed immune reconstitution syndrome. The immune response to current opportunistic infections may result in the need for additional treatment. Autoimmune disorders have also been reported as part of immune reconstitution syndrome.

Nucleoside analogues, including FTC and TDF, have been associated with lactic acidosis and severe hepatomegaly with steatosis. Some cases have been fatal. Treatment with FTC/TDF should be discontinued for any individual with laboratory or clinical findings of hepatotoxicity or lactic acidosis.

Side Effects
Depression, diarrhea, dizziness, fatigue, headache, insomnia, nausea, rashes

Drug–Drug Interactions
FTC/TDF is excreted primarily by the kidneys. Co-administration of FTC/TDF with other drugs that are eliminated by active tubular secretion may increase concentrations of FTC/TDF. Examples include acyclovir, adefovir dipivoxil, cidofovir, ganciclovir, valacyclovir, valganciclovir, aminoglycosides such as gentamicin, and high-dose or multiple nonsteroidal anti-inflammatory drugs (NSAIDs).

Hepatitis C antiviral medications such as ledipasvir/sofosbuvir, sofosbuvir/velpatasvir, and sofosbuvir/velpatasvir/voxilaprevir may increase levels of tenofovir disoproxil fumarate.

HIV-1 protease inhibitors atazanavir/ritonavir, darunavir/ritonavir, and lopinavir/ritonavir may increase levels of tenofovir disoproxil fumarate.

FTC/TDF may increase the concentration of the nucleoside reverse transcriptase inhibitor didanosine.

Specific Considerations for Women
Pregnancy
Antiretroviral therapy should be provided during pregnancy for all women who are HIV-positive, to minimize the risk of perinatal transmission. For women at risk of acquiring HIV-1, consideration should be given to continuing or initiating FTC/TDF for HIV-1 PrEP during pregnancy as part of an overall HIV risk reduction strategy. There is no indication that FTC/TDF exposure during pregnancy increases the overall risk of major birth defects when compared to the 2.7% background rate among pregnant women in the United States.

Healthcare providers are encouraged to report cases of antenatal antiretroviral drug exposure to the Antiretroviral Pregnancy Registry. The registry can be contacted by telephone 800-258-4263 or fax 800-800-1052. The Antiretroviral Pregnancy Registry is also accessible via the Internet at http://www.apregistry.com.

Breastfeeding
To reduce the risk of postnatal transmission, women in the United States who are HIV-positive are advised by the Centers for Disease Control and Prevention to avoid breastfeeding, regardless of antiretroviral treatment. Limited data suggest that small amounts of emtricitabine and tenofovir are excreted into breast milk.

Adolescent women
The Food and Drug Administration has expanded the use of FTC/TDF for PrEP for adolescents who weigh at least 35 kg (77 lb).

Elderly women
Data are lacking on whether age-related dose adjustments are necessary for women over the age of 65.

Dose
HIV-1 pre-exposure prophylaxis (PrEP):
Recommended dose for adults who are HIV-1 negative and adolescents weighing at least 35 kg (77 lb): One FTC/TDF tablet at a fixed dose of 200 mg of FTC and 300 mg of TDF orally once daily with or without food.

Treatment of HIV-1 infection:
Recommended dose for adults and children weighing at least 35 kg (77 lb): One FTC/TDF tablet (containing 200 mg of FTC and 300 mg of TDF) orally once daily with or without food.

How Supplied
FTC/TDF is supplied in 4 different fixed doses for oral use:
   100 mg of FTC and 150 mg of TDF
   133 mg of FTC and 200 mg of TDF
   167 mg of FTC and 250 mg of TDF
   200 mg of FTC and 300 mg of TDF

Prescribing Considerations

FTC/TDF has a **black box warning** for increased drug resistance if used for PrEP by individuals who are HIV-positive, and for acute exacerbations of HBV after discontinuation of the medication for individuals who have HBV. FTC/TDF for PrEP must only be prescribed for individuals who are HIV-1 negative, and HIV-negative status must be confirmed immediately prior to beginning the medication and at 3-month intervals during treatment. HIV testing should also be performed with the diagnosis of another sexually transmitted infection (STI). Individuals with HBV infection who are taking FTC/TDF should be monitored closely with laboratory testing and clinical examinations for several months after discontinuing FTC/TDF.

Testing for HIV and HBV is necessary immediately prior to beginning FTC/TDF. Individuals who have not been vaccinated for HBV should be offered vaccination prior to treatment.

HIV-1 antibodies may not be detectable during the acute phase of infection. Individuals with seronegative testing should be evaluated for recent (past one month) symptoms of acute HIV viral infection such as fever, chills, myalgia, fatigue, and skin rashes. If symptoms are present or potential recent exposure has occurred in the past month (unprotected sex, condom break, blood or body fluid exposure to an individual with known HIV-1), FTC/TDF for PrEP should be delayed for one month to confirm HIV-1 negative status.

FTC/TDF should be used only as one part of a comprehensive plan to reduce the risk of HIV acquisition. Other sexual risk reduction behaviors, such as use of condoms, limiting partners, knowing HIV status of partners, viral suppression of partners who are HIV-positive, and testing and treatment of other STIs that can facilitate HIV-1 transmission should be discussed.

Adherence to daily dosing for PrEP is important. The efficacy of FTC/TDF in preventing HIV-1 infection is correlated with adherence to treatment that results in consistent drug levels.

Due to the possibility of adverse renal function associated with tenofovir disoproxil fumarate, serum creatinine, estimated creatinine clearance, urine glucose, and urine protein should be assessed prior to initiating and during treatment with FTC/TDF.

The effects of BMD changes on long-term bone health and future fracture risk among women taking tenofovir disoproxil fumarate are unknown. Assessment of BMD should be considered for women based on age, history of fracture, and other risk factors for osteoporosis or bone loss. It is not known if supplementation with calcium and vitamin D is beneficial.

Cost: $$$$$

Erythromycin (Ery-tab, E.E.S. 400, E-Mycin, and others)

E

Therapeutic class: Antibiotic

Chemical class: Macrolide

Indications
Erythromycin is used to treat a broad range of infections caused by susceptible strains of bacteria such as *Streptococcus pyogenes, S. pneumoniae, Listeria monocytogenes, Mycoplasma pneumoniae, Neisseria gonorrhoeae, Chlamydia trachomatis,* and *Bordetella pertussis.*

Contraindications
Erythromycin is contraindicated for individuals with a known allergic reaction or hypersensitivity to the drug. It is also contraindicated for use with the following medications: astemizole, cisapride, dihydroergotamine, ergotamine, pimozide, and terfenadine.

Mechanism of Action
Erythromycin inhibits protein synthesis by binding 50S ribosomal subunits of susceptible organisms.

Metabolism & Excretion
Hepatic and biliary

Adverse Reactions
Hepatic toxicity has occurred. Allergic reactions and hearing loss have been reported with erythromycin.

Clostridium difficile-associated diarrhea (CDAD) has been reported with the use of antibiotics, including erythromycin.

Side Effects
Gastrointestinal (GI) upset including abdominal pain, anorexia, diarrhea, nausea, and vomiting. Overgrowth of fungi can result in oral thrush and vulvovaginal candidiasis.

Drug–Drug Interactions
In addition to the contraindications listed earlier, severe adverse reactions (hypotension, rhabdomyolysis, toxicity) have occurred when erythromycin is taken concomitantly with CYP3A4 substrates, including amlodipine, atorvastatin, colchicine, diltiazem, lovastatin, simvastatin, and verapamil.

Erythromycin may increase digoxin and theophylline levels and reduce the clearance of benzodiazepines.

Erythromycin may prolong the effects of oral anticoagulants.

Other drug–drug interactions are possible. The full prescribing information should be consulted.

Specific Considerations for Women
Pregnancy
Erythromycin can be taken during pregnancy.

Breastfeeding
Erythromycin is excreted in breast milk in low levels and can be given directly to infants. Erythromycin is acceptable for women who are breastfeeding. Adverse reactions for the infant are rare, but GI effects such as diarrhea and thrush are possible.

Adolescent women
Erythromycin can be used by adolescent women.

Elderly women
Individuals who are older can take erythromycin but are more susceptible to cardiac arrhythmias, erythromycin-related hearing loss, and increased effects on oral anticoagulants than younger individuals.

Dose
Dosing is variable and dependent on the wide range of infections that can be treated with erythromycin. In general, erythromycin is given orally either three or four times per day. Consult full prescribing information for specific dose amounts.

How Supplied
Erythromycin is available as 250-mg, 333-mg, 400-mg, and 500-mg tablets for oral use.

E

Prescribing Considerations
GI upset is common. Although absorption is enhanced on an empty stomach, taking erythromycin with food may decrease GI symptoms.

The entire course of medication should be finished even if symptoms resolve.

There are many drug–drug interactions. A complete medication history should be taken prior to prescribing erythromycin.

Cost: $

Estrogen (Climara, Estrasorb, Evamist, Femring, Premarin, Vivelle-Dot, and others)
Estrogen plus progesterone (Activella, FemHrt, Premphase, Prempro, and others)

Therapeutic class: Hormone replacement

Chemical class: Estrogen, estrogen + progestin

Indications
Estrogen or estrogen + progesterone is indicated for moderate to severe vasomotor symptoms (VMS) of menopause and vulvovaginal atrophy due to menopause.

Contraindications

Per package labeling, estrogen is contraindicated with:

1. Undiagnosed abnormal vaginal bleeding
2. Known, suspected, or history of breast cancer
3. Known or suspected estrogen-dependent neoplasia
4. Active deep vein thrombosis (DVT), pulmonary embolism (PE), or a history of these conditions
5. Active arterial thromboembolic disease or cardiovascular disease (CVD) such as myocardial infarction (MI) or stroke, or a history of these conditions
6. Known anaphylactic reaction or angioedema to estrogens or progestins
7. Known liver dysfunction or disease
8. Known protein C, protein S, or antithrombin deficiency or other known thrombophilic disorders
9. Known or suspected pregnancy

Mechanism of Action

Estrogens act through binding to nuclear receptors in estrogen-responsive tissues.

Metabolism & Excretion

Hepatic and renal

Adverse Reactions

Most noted adverse reactions are associated with systemic absorption of oral estrogen. Route of administration, dose, and length of treatment should be considered when evaluating a woman's individual risk for serious adverse events.

Estrogens increase the risk for breast and ovarian neoplasia, cholecystitis, DVT, hypercalcemia, hypothyroidism, MI, PE, and stroke. Estrogen use has been linked to dementia for women over age 65.

Unopposed estrogen for women with an *intact uterus* is associated with endometrial hyperplasia and the risk of endometrial carcinoma.

Estrogens may cause elevations in blood pressure and cholesterol.

Side Effects
Breast enlargement, breast pain, headache, leg cramps, leukorrhea, pelvic pain, vaginal bleeding, vaginitis, vasodilation

Drug–Drug Interactions
Inhibitors of CYP3A4, such as clarithromycin, erythromycin, grapefruit juice, itraconazole, ketoconazole, and ritonavir may increase plasma concentrations of estrogens and may result in side effects.

Inducers of CYP3A4, such as carbamazepine, phenobarbital, rifampin, and St. John's wort, may reduce plasma concentrations of estrogens. This could possibly lessen therapeutic effects and/or cause changes in the uterine bleeding profile.

Aminoglutethimide administered concomitantly with medroxyprogesterone acetate (MPA) may significantly depress the bioavailability of MPA.

Specific Considerations for Women
Pregnancy
Systemic estrogen alone or estrogen plus progesterone is contraindicated during pregnancy. No increase in birth defects has been noted for infants inadvertently exposed to estrogen or estrogen plus progesterone, but pregnancy is not a condition in which these medications as hormone therapy for VMS of menopause would provide any therapeutic effect.

Breastfeeding
The route of administration and dose of hormone therapy influence the amount transferred into breast milk. Oral and vaginal administration result in measurable amounts in breast milk, but transdermal patches do not. Because exposure for the infant is possible, estrogen alone or estrogen plus progesterone should not be used during lactation. Water-soluble lubricants can be considered for breastfeeding-associated dyspareunia, and nonhormonal methods can be considered if VMS occur during lactation.

Adolescent women
Atrophic vaginitis, VMS of menopause, and vulvovaginal atrophy are not conditions associated with adolescence.

Elderly women

Systemic hormone therapy is indicated for postmenopausal vulvovaginal atrophy and VMS of perimenopause and menopause. It is appropriate for use by women who are postmenopausal. A possible increase in the risk of dementia for women over age 65 has been reported.

Dose

Dose is variable and dependent on the brand, formulation, and delivery system chosen. Consult full prescribing information for each medication.

How Supplied

Systemic hormone therapy is available as pills, transdermal patches, vaginal rings, and topical skin preparations. Consult full prescribing information for each medication.

Prescribing Considerations

All estrogen preparations have a **black box warning** to highlight:

1. Risk of endometrial cancer for women with an intact uterus who use unopposed estrogen
2. Estrogen is inappropriate for the prevention of CVD or dementia
3. Estrogen increases the risk of DVT, MI, PE, and stroke
4. Possible increased risk of dementia for women over age 65 who use estrogen

For women with an intact uterus, adding a progestin will decrease the risk of endometrial hyperplasia from unopposed estrogen. Systemic hormone therapy is available in estrogen-alone or estrogen-plus-progesterone formulations.

The lowest effective dose for the shortest duration is prudent.

Abnormal vaginal bleeding should be reported to a healthcare provider and investigated appropriately.

Abrupt withdrawal of estrogen for the treatment of VMS of menopause may result in the onset of new VMS. Reducing the dose slowly can be considered if women are concerned about VMS.

Vaginal preparations should be considered if atrophic vaginitis, dyspareunia, and vulvovaginal atrophy are the primary conditions.

Cost: $–$$$

Estrogen plus progesterone combined hormonal contraception (CHC): pills/patch/ring

Oral contraceptive pills: Many individual brands

Xulane contraceptive patch

NuvaRing vaginal contraceptive ring

Annovera vaginal contraceptive ring (approved)

Therapeutic class: Contraceptive

Chemical class: Hormones

Indications
CHC, in any formulation and delivery system, is indicated for the prevention of pregnancy.

Some brands of combined oral contraceptive pills have an indication for acne treatment if the woman also desires oral contraception.

CHC has also been used off label in the management of abnormal uterine bleeding, amenorrhea, dysmenorrhea, endometriosis, heavy menstrual bleeding, and menstrual cycle control.

Contraindications
CHC is contraindicated for women with:

1. Thrombophlebitis or thromboembolic disorders
2. History of deep vein thrombophlebitis (DVT)
3. Cerebral vascular or coronary artery disease
4. Known or suspected carcinoma of the breast
5. Carcinoma of the endometrium or other known or suspected estrogen-dependent neoplasia
6. Undiagnosed abnormal vaginal bleeding
7. Cholestatic jaundice of pregnancy or jaundice with prior use
8. Hepatic adenomas or carcinomas
9. Known or suspected pregnancy

10. Known hypersensitivity to CHC
11. Receiving hepatitis C drug combinations containing ombitasvir/paritaprevir/ritonavir, with or without dasabuvir, due to the potential for liver enzyme elevations

Mechanism of Action
The primary mechanism of action is inhibition of follicular development and prevention of ovulation. CHCs may also thicken the cervical mucus and alter the endometrium to interfere with implantation.

Metabolism & Excretion
Hepatic and renal

Adverse Reactions
The most serious adverse reactions are venous thrombotic events (VTEs), including cerebral vascular accidents (CVAs), DVT, and myocardial infarction (MI). Other potentially serious events include abnormal carbohydrate metabolism, abnormal liver function, depression, gallbladder disease, hypertension, and liver tumors. Rare cases of toxic shock syndrome have occurred with the vaginal ring.

Side Effects
Breast tenderness, chloasma, headache, irregular menstrual bleeding and spotting, nausea
    Local skin reactions have been reported with the contraceptive patch.

Drug–Drug Interactions
Drugs or herbal products that induce certain enzymes, such as CYP3A4, may decrease the effectiveness of CHCs or increase breakthrough bleeding. These include, but are not limited to, carbamazepine, phenobarbital, rifampin, and St. John's wort.
    Concomitant administration of strong or moderate CYP3A4 inhibitors such as fluconazole, grapefruit juice, itraconazole, ketoconazole, or voriconazole may increase plasma estrogen and/or progestin concentrations.

Specific Considerations for Women
Pregnancy
CHC is indicated for the prevention of pregnancy and therefore has no therapeutic benefit for women who are pregnant. However, if a woman becomes pregnant while taking CHC, there doesn't appear to be an increased risk of birth defects for fetuses exposed to CHC. Once the pregnancy is discovered, CHC should be stopped.

Breastfeeding
Estrogen during lactation has been linked to a decreased quantity and quality of breast milk. Women who are breastfeeding and require contraception should consider a progestin-only or nonhormonal method.

Adolescent women
Adolescent women who require contraception may use CHC.

Elderly women
Women who are postmenopausal are not at risk for pregnancy, and therefore CHC provides no therapeutic benefit.

Dose: Variable, depending on formulation
Combined oral contraceptive pills:
One pill orally every day per product-specific directions. Combined oral contraceptive pills are available in a range of doses and formulations.

Estrogen doses range from 10 mcg to 50 mcg of ethinyl estradiol.

Progestins include desogestrel, drospirenone, ethynodiol diacetate, levonorgestrel, norethindrone, norgestimate, norgestrel in varying doses.

Vaginal contraceptive ring (NuvaRing):
Contains a total of 11.7 mg etonogestrel and 2.7 mg ethinyl estradiol that is released over 3 weeks. One ring inserted vaginally for 3 weeks, then one ring-free week. The next week is started with a new ring.

Vaginal contraceptive ring (Annovera):
Contains 103 mg segesterone acetate and 17.4 mg ethinyl estradiol. The ring releases an average of 0.15 mg/day of segesterone acetate and 0.013 mg/day

of ethinyl estradiol. One ring inserted vaginally for 3 weeks, then one ring-free week. The same ring can be used for a full year. Availability expected in 2020.

Contraceptive patch (Xulane):
Releases 150 mcg/day norelgestromin and 35 mcg/day ethinyl estradiol. One patch is worn for a week and replaced with a new patch each week for 3 weeks, then one patch-free week.

How Supplied
Combined oral contraceptive pills are supplied as a single pack for one-month or three-month use.

The vaginal contraceptive ring (NuvaRing) is supplied as a single ring for one-month use.

The vaginal contraceptive ring (Annovera) is supplied as a single ring for 12 months of use.

The contraceptive patch (Xulane) is supplied as a box containing 3 patches for one-month use.

Prescribing Considerations
All forms of CHC have a **black box warning** for the increased risk of severe and possibly fatal cardiovascular events when used with cigarette smoking, especially for women over the age of 35. Additionally, the contraceptive patch may result in higher levels of estrogen than oral contraceptives, which could further increase the risk of VTEs. Women over the age of 35 who smoke should not use CHC, and all women who wish to use CHC should be advised not to smoke.

Despite information contained in some antibiotic product labeling and dispensed by some pharmacies, recent evidence **does not** support a link between nonrifampin antibiotics and hormonal contraception failure.

Each formulation and delivery system has specific instructions for use that should be referred to prior to prescribing, including instructions on how to manage missed or late doses of CHC and how and when to transition between different contraceptive methods.

Adherence to correct use significantly increases the effectiveness of CHC.

CHC can be initiated on the first day of the menstrual cycle or at any point in the menstrual cycle if it is reasonably certain the woman is not pregnant.

CHC may raise blood pressure in some women. It is prudent to assess blood pressure within 3 months of initiating CHC and yearly thereafter.

Data are conflicting about the effect of body weight (overweight and obesity) on the effectiveness of CHC. Package labeling specifies that the contraceptive patch may be less effective for women who weigh more than 90 kg (198 lb). There is emerging evidence that oral CHC may be less effective for women who are obese, but data are conflicting. The CDC U.S. Medical Eligibility Criteria for Contraceptive Use lists all forms of CHC as either a category 1 or 2 recommendation for women with a body mass index (BMI) greater than 30 kg/m^2.

New and emerging data suggest that some women may have a genetic mutation that results in increased metabolism of the hormones in CHC, possibly placing them at a greater risk for contraceptive failure. How this may affect clinical practice and contraceptive counseling is not known.

In general, CHC should be stopped 2 weeks prior to surgery with immobilization and not be restarted until 2 weeks after surgery if mobility will be significantly restricted.

Cost: $–$$$$

Estrogen vaginal cream/tablets/ring (Estrace, Estring, Premarin, Vagifem)

Therapeutic class: Estrogen replacement

Chemical class: Estrogen

Indications
Estrogen vaginal cream is indicated for the treatment of atrophic vaginitis and dyspareunia associated with vulvovaginal atrophy of menopause.

Estrogen vaginal tablets and the vaginal ring (Estring) are indicated for the treatment of atrophic vaginitis due to menopause.

Contraindications

Per package labeling, vaginal estrogen is contraindicated with:

1. Undiagnosed abnormal vaginal bleeding
2. Known, suspected, or history of breast cancer
3. Known or suspected estrogen-dependent neoplasia
4. Active deep vein thrombosis (DVT), pulmonary embolism (PE), or a history of these conditions
5. Active arterial thromboembolic disease or cardiovascular disease (CVD) such as stroke or myocardial infarction (MI), or a history of these conditions
6. Known anaphylactic reaction or angioedema to estrogens or estrogen cream/tablets
7. Known liver dysfunction or disease
8. Known protein C, protein S, or antithrombin deficiency or other known thrombophilic disorders
9. Known or suspected pregnancy

Mechanism of Action

Estrogens act through binding to nuclear receptors in estrogen-responsive tissues.

Metabolism & Excretion

Hepatic and renal

Adverse Reactions

Most noted adverse reactions are associated with systemic absorption of oral estrogen. Vaginal estrogen, in smaller doses to treat vulvovaginal atrophy, is systemically absorbed but to a lesser extent than oral estrogen. Route of administration, dose, and length of treatment should be considered when evaluating a woman's individual risk for serious adverse events.

Estrogens increase the risk for cholecystitis, DVT, hypercalcemia, hypothyroidism, MI, PE, and stroke, and may increase the risk of breast and ovarian neoplasia. Estrogen use has been linked to dementia among women over age 65.

Unopposed estrogen taken by women with an *intact uterus* is associated with endometrial hyperplasia and the risk of endometrial carcinoma.

Estrogens may cause elevations in blood pressure and cholesterol.

Side Effects

Vaginal estrogen preparations may cause breast pain, headache, leukorrhea, pelvic pain, vaginal bleeding, vaginitis, and vasodilation.

Drug–Drug Interactions

Inhibitors of CYP3A4, such as clarithromycin, erythromycin, grapefruit juice, itraconazole, ketoconazole, and ritonavir may increase plasma concentrations of estrogens and may result in side effects.

Inducers of CYP3A4, such as carbamazepine, phenobarbital, rifampin, and St. John's wort, may reduce plasma concentrations of estrogens. This could possibly result in lessened therapeutic effects.

Specific Considerations for Women

Pregnancy

Vaginal estrogen is contraindicated during pregnancy. No increase in birth defects has been noted for infants inadvertently exposed to estrogen, but pregnancy is not a condition in which vaginal estrogen would provide any therapeutic effect.

Breastfeeding

Vaginal administration of estrogen results in measurable levels in breast milk, although the concentration is variable. Because infant exposure is possible, vaginal estrogen should not be used during lactation. Water-soluble lubricants can be considered for breastfeeding-associated vulvovaginal atrophy and dyspareunia.

Adolescent women

Atrophic vaginitis and vulvovaginal atrophy are not conditions associated with adolescence and vaginal estrogen use has not been studied in the pediatric population.

Elderly women
Vaginal administration is indicated for postmenopausal vulvovaginal atrophy.
It is appropriate for use by women who are postmenopausal.

Dose
Each gram of vaginal cream contains 0.625 mg of conjugated estrogens. For
vaginal cream, 0.5 grams is the usual starting dose.

Estrogen vaginal tablets are available in 10 mcg and 25 mcg of estrogen
per tablet. For vaginal tablets, the usual starting dose is 10 mcg.

The vaginal ring (Estring) contains a total of 2 mg of estradiol that is
released slowly over the course of 90 days.

Atrophic vaginitis:
Estrogen cream is administered intravaginally each night for 21 days with a
7-day break. This cycle can be repeated as needed based on response. The
dose can be increased to 2 grams nightly if there is an inadequate response
to lower doses.

Estrogen tablets: 1 tablet is inserted intravaginally each day for 2 weeks,
followed by 1 tablet twice weekly (for example, Monday and Thursday or
Tuesday and Friday).

Estrogen ring (Estring): One ring is inserted into the upper third of the
vaginal canal and left in place for 90 days. It is replaced with a new ring if
continued treatment is needed after 90 days.

Dyspareunia associated with menopause:
Estrogen cream is administered intravaginally each night for 21 days with
a 7-day break. An alternative regimen is twice-weekly administration (for
example, Monday and Thursday or Tuesday and Friday).

How Supplied
Estrogen vaginal cream is supplied as a 30-gram tube of medication with
applicators.

Estrogen vaginal tablets are supplied in cartons with 8 or 18 single-use
applicators.

Estrogen vaginal ring (Estring) is supplied as a single ring containing
2 mg of estradiol in a sealed pouch.

Prescribing Considerations

Vaginal estrogen preparations have a **black box warning** to highlight:

1. Risk of endometrial cancer for women with an intact uterus who use unopposed estrogen
2. Inappropriateness of estrogen use for the prevention of CVD or dementia
3. Estrogen increases the risk of DVT, MI, PE, and stroke
4. Possible increased risk of dementia for women over 65 who use estrogen

For women with an intact uterus, adding a progestin can be considered based on length of treatment and dose of estrogen used.

The lowest effective dose for the shortest duration is prudent. Number of applications per week and length of treatment can be adjusted based on response.

Abnormal vaginal bleeding should be reported to a healthcare provider and investigated appropriately.

There are 2 brands of vaginal rings available with similar names but different doses and indications. Estring contains 2 mg of estradiol and is indicated for the treatment of moderate to severe symptoms of vulvovaginal atrophy. Femring is available in 2 different doses that release either 0.05 mg/day or 0.1 mg/day of estradiol and is indicated for the treatment of vasomotor symptoms of menopause and vulvovaginal atrophy. Prescribers need to be cautious when choosing the correct dose and indication.

The vaginal ring need not be removed during intercourse.

Cost: $–$$$

Estrogen/bazedoxifene (Duavee)

Therapeutic class: Hormone replacement

Chemical class: Estrogen + estrogen agonist/antagonist

Indications

Indicated for moderate to severe vasomotor symptoms (VMS) of menopause and prevention of postmenopausal osteoporosis.

Contraindications

Per package labeling, estrogen is contraindicated with:

1. Undiagnosed abnormal vaginal bleeding
2. Known, suspected, or history of breast cancer
3. Known or suspected estrogen-dependent neoplasia
4. Active deep vein thrombosis (DVT), pulmonary embolism (PE), or a history of these conditions
5. Active arterial thromboembolic disease or cardiovascular disease (CVD) such as myocardial infarction (MI) or stroke, or a history of these conditions
6. Known anaphylactic reaction or angioedema to estrogens or bazedoxifene
7. Known liver dysfunction or disease
8. Known protein C, protein S, or antithrombin deficiency or other known thrombophilic disorders
9. Known or suspected pregnancy

Mechanism of Action

Estrogens act through binding to nuclear receptors in estrogen-responsive tissues. Bazedoxifene is an estrogen agonist/antagonist that acts as an agonist in some estrogen-sensitive tissues and an antagonist in others, such as the uterus. Bazedoxifene reduces the risk of endometrial hyperplasia that can occur with the use of estrogen alone.

Metabolism & Excretion

Hepatic and renal

Adverse Reactions

Most noted adverse reactions are associated with systemic absorption of oral estrogen. Route of administration, dose, and length of treatment should be considered when evaluating a woman's individual risk for serious adverse events.

Estrogen increases the risk for breast and ovarian neoplasia, cholecystitis, DVT, hypercalcemia, hypothyroidism, MI, PE, and stroke. Estrogen use has been linked to dementia for women over age 65.

Unopposed estrogen for women with an *intact uterus* is associated with endometrial hyperplasia and the risk of endometrial carcinoma.

Estrogens may cause elevations in blood pressure and cholesterol.

Side Effects

Abdominal pain, breast pain, diarrhea, dyspepsia, headache, muscle spasms/pain, nausea, vaginal bleeding, vaginitis

Drug–Drug Interactions

Inhibitors of CYP3A4, such as clarithromycin, erythromycin, grapefruit juice, itraconazole, ketoconazole, and ritonavir may increase plasma concentrations of estrogens and may result in side effects.

Inducers of CYP3A4, such as carbamazepine, phenobarbital, rifampin, and St. John's wort may reduce plasma concentrations of estrogens. This could possibly lessen therapeutic effects and/or cause changes in the uterine bleeding profile.

Bazedoxifene undergoes metabolism by uridine diphosphate glucuronosyltransferase (UGT) enzymes in the intestinal tract and liver. The metabolism of bazedoxifene may be increased by concomitant use of substances known to induce UGTs, such as carbamazepine, phenobarbital, phenytoin, and rifampin. A reduction in bazedoxifene exposure may be associated with an increased risk of endometrial hyperplasia.

Specific Considerations for Women

Pregnancy

Systemic estrogen alone or estrogen plus bazedoxifene is contraindicated during pregnancy. No increase in birth defects has been noted for infants inadvertently exposed to estrogen, but pregnancy is not a condition in which these medications as hormone therapy for VMS of menopause would provide any therapeutic effect.

Breastfeeding

The route of administration and dose of hormone therapy influence the amount transferred into breast milk. Oral administration results in measurable amounts in breast milk and may decrease the quantity and quality of breast milk. There is no information on bazedoxifene during lactation.

Because exposure to the infant is possible, estrogen/bazedoxifene should not be used during lactation. Water-soluble lubricants can be considered for breastfeeding-associated dyspareunia, and nonhormonal methods can be considered if VMS occur during lactation.

Adolescent women
Atrophic vaginitis, VMS of menopause, and vulvovaginal atrophy are not conditions associated with adolescence.

Elderly women
Systemic hormone replacement is indicated for women who are postmenopausal and experiencing vulvovaginal atrophy and/or VMS of menopause. A possible increase in the risk of dementia for women over age 65 has been reported. This medication has not been studied for women over age 75 and is not recommended for this age group.

Dose
The dose is a combination tablet containing conjugated estrogens 0.45 mg and bazedoxifene 20 mg. One tablet is taken orally every day.

How Supplied
A single combination tablet for oral use containing conjugated estrogens 0.45 mg and bazedoxifene 20 mg in 2 blister packages of 15 tablets each

Prescribing Considerations
All estrogen preparations have a **black box warning** to highlight:

1. Risk of endometrial cancer for women with an intact uterus who use unopposed estrogen
2. That estrogen is inappropriate for the prevention of CVD or dementia
3. That estrogen increases the risk of DVT, MI, PE, and stroke
4. Possible increased risk of dementia for women over 65 who use estrogen

   Women taking estrogen/bazedoxifene should not take additional estrogen, estrogen agonists/antagonists, or progesterone. The lowest effective dose for the shortest duration is prudent.

   Systemic exposure of estrogen/bazedoxifene may be lower for women with a body mass index (BMI) greater than 30 kg/m^2.

The pharmacokinetics of estrogen/bazedoxifene have not been evaluated for women with renal or hepatic impairment.

Abnormal vaginal bleeding should be reported to a healthcare provider and investigated appropriately.

Abrupt withdrawal of estrogen for the treatment of VMS of menopause may result in the onset of new VMS. Reducing the dose slowly can be considered if women are concerned about VMS.

Vaginal preparations should be considered if atrophic vaginitis, dyspareunia, and vulvovaginal atrophy are the primary conditions.

Estrogen-containing medications should not be used for the prevention of osteoporosis without VMS of menopause. Nonestrogen-containing medication should be considered first for prevention of osteoporosis.

Calcium and vitamin D should be considered if there is a dietary deficiency.

Cost: $$$$

Etonogestrel implant (Nexplanon)

Therapeutic class: Contraceptive

Chemical class: Progestin

Indications
The etonogestrel implant is indicated for the prevention of pregnancy for up to 3 years.

Contraindications
The etonogestrel implant is contraindicated with:

1. Known or suspected pregnancy
2. Current or history of thrombosis or thromboembolic disorders
3. Liver tumors, benign or malignant, or active liver disease
4. Undiagnosed abnormal vaginal bleeding
5. Known or suspected breast cancer, personal history of breast cancer, or other progestin-sensitive cancer, now or in the past
6. Allergic reaction to etonogestrel or any of the components of the implant

Mechanism of Action
Prevention of pregnancy is achieved through suppression of ovulation, increased viscosity of the cervical mucus, and alterations in the endometrium.

Metabolism & Excretion
Hepatic and renal

Adverse Reactions
Insertion or removal complications, including a broken or bent implant, can occur.

Ectopic pregnancy is uncommon among women who use the etonogestrel implant, but a pregnancy that occurs with the implant in place has a higher risk of an extrauterine placement.

There have been postmarketing reports of venous thrombotic events.

Side Effects
Abdominal pain, acne, breast pain, change in menstrual bleeding pattern, headache, mood changes, pain at insertion/removal site, vaginitis, weight increase

Drug–Drug Interactions
Drugs or herbal products that induce certain enzymes, including cytochrome CYP3A4, may decrease the plasma concentrations of etonogestrel. This could diminish the implant's effectiveness or increase irregular bleeding.

Co-administration with a strong or moderate CYP3A4 inhibitor such as fluconazole, grapefruit juice, itraconazole, ketoconazole, or voriconazole may increase the serum concentrations of progestins, including etonogestrel.

Significant changes (increase or decrease) in the plasma concentrations of progestin have been noted with co-administration of HIV protease inhibitors and hepatitis C (HCV) protease inhibitors.

Specific Considerations for Women
Pregnancy
The etonogestrel implant is indicated for the prevention of pregnancy and therefore provides no therapeutic benefit for women who are pregnant. There are no data that suggest an increased risk of birth defects for infants

inadvertently exposed to etonogestrel in early pregnancy. If a pregnancy is recognized with the etonogestrel implant in place, the implant should be removed if the pregnancy is continued.

Breastfeeding
The etonogestrel implant is acceptable for women who are breastfeeding. According to the U.S. Medical Eligibility Criteria for Contraceptive Use, it is a category 1 or 2 recommendation and can be inserted immediately post-partum or postabortion. The quantity and quality of breast milk and infant growth do not appear to be adversely affected.

Adolescent women
Adolescent women may use the etonogestrel implant.

Elderly women
Women who are postmenopausal are not at risk for pregnancy, and therefore the etonogestrel implant provides no therapeutic benefit.

Dose
One 68-mg etonogestrel implant is inserted subdermally just under the skin at the inner side of the nondominant upper arm. The implant can remain in place for 3 years.

How Supplied
The etonogestrel implant is supplied as a single, radiopaque, rod-shaped implant, containing 68 mg etonogestrel, preloaded in the needle of a disposable applicator.

Prescribing Considerations
All healthcare providers should receive training in the insertion and removal of the etonogestrel implant. Additionally, package labeling provides detailed instructions.

The implant should be removed at the end of 3 years of use. If continued contraception is desired, a new implant can be inserted on the same day as removal along the same tract. Emerging research has suggested that the implant may be effective for longer than the 3-year Food and Drug

Administration (FDA) approval. Providers should remain current with new research and changes in use.

If the implant is inserted between days 1 and 5 of the menstrual cycle, no backup contraception is needed. If inserted at another time during the menstrual cycle, pregnancy should first be excluded, and backup contraception is required for the next 7 days.

According to product labeling, serum concentrations of etonogestrel are inversely related to body weight and decrease with time after implant insertion. The product labeling highlights the possibility that the etonogestrel implant may be less effective for women with a body mass index (BMI) in the overweight or obese category. However, newer research does not support a relationship between body weight and decreased efficacy. U.S. Medical Eligibility Criteria for Contraceptive Use lists the implant as a category 1 recommendation for women with a BMI greater than or equal to 30 kg/m^2.

Irregular and unscheduled bleeding are common. Women should be counseled regarding the expected changes in the menstrual cycle.

Cost: $$$$$

Flibanserin (Addyi)

Therapeutic class: Sexual dysfunction agent

Chemical class: Multifunctional serotonin agonist antagonist (MSAA)

Indications
Flibanserin is indicated for the treatment of hypoactive sexual desire disorder (HSDD) for women who are premenopausal. HSDD is characterized by low sexual desire that causes marked distress or interpersonal difficulty and is not due to (1) co-existing medical or psychiatric condition, (2) interpersonal relationship issues, or (3) side effects from other medications or substances.

Contraindications
Main contraindications include concomitant use with moderate or strong CYP3A4 inhibitors and hepatic impairment.

Mechanism of Action
The exact mechanism of action in the treatment of HSDD is not known. Flibanserin has a high affinity for serotonin receptors. It may improve sexual functioning by enhancing the release of dopamine and norepinephrine while reducing serotonin release in areas of the brain that mediate symptoms of reduced sexual interest and desire.

Metabolism & Excretion
Hepatic and renal

Adverse Reactions
Significant adverse reactions include the possibility of central nervous system (CNS) impairment (somnolence), hypotension, and syncope.

Side Effects
Dizziness, drowsiness, fatigue, nausea

Major Interactions
Moderate to strong CYP3A4 inhibitors increase flibanserin concentrations, which can potentiate CNS depression, hypotension, and syncope. These include amprenavir, atazanavir, boceprevir, ciprofloxacin, clarithromycin, conivaptan, diltiazem, erythromycin, fluconazole, fosamprenavir, grapefruit juice, indinavir, itraconazole, ketoconazole, nefazodone, nelfinavir, posaconazole, ritonavir, saquinavir, telaprevir, telithromycin, and verapamil.

Multiple weak CYP3A4 inhibitors could potentially increase flibanserin concentrations and increase the risk of CNS depression, hypotension, and syncope. These include cimetidine, combined oral contraceptives, fluoxetine, ginkgo, and ranitidine.

Strong CYP2C19 inhibitors could potentially increase flibanserin concentrations and increase the risk of CNS depression, hypotension, and syncope. These include antifungals, benzodiazepines, proton pump inhibitors (PPIs), and selective serotonin reuptake inhibitors (SSRIs).

CYP3A4 inducers substantially decrease flibanserin exposure and reduce effectiveness. These include carbamazepine, phenobarbital, phenytoin, rifabutin, rifampin, rifapetine, and St. John's wort.

Flibanserin increases digoxin levels, which could lead to toxicity.

Other CNS depressants may increase the risk of CNS impairment and somnolence. These include benzodiazepines, diphenhydramine, hypnotics, and opioids.

Specific Considerations for Women
Pregnancy
There have been no studies of flibanserin use by women who are pregnant, and flibanserin is not indicated during pregnancy. If a woman becomes pregnant while taking flibanserin, she should stop the medication and notify her healthcare provider.

Breastfeeding
It is unknown if flibanserin is excreted in breast milk or if there are any potential effects on an infant who is breastfeeding. Therefore, flibanserin should not be used by women who are breastfeeding.

Adolescent women
Flibanserin has not been evaluated among the adolescent population.

Elderly women
Flibanserin is not indicated for women who are postmenopausal and have HSDD. Use among postmenopausal women has not been evaluated.

Dose
The recommended dose is 100 mg orally each day, taken at bedtime.

How Supplied
Flibanserin is supplied as a 100-mg tablet for oral use.

Prescribing Considerations
Flibanserin has a **black box warning** for hypotension, interaction with alcohol, and syncope; use with moderate to strong CYP3A4 inhibitors; and use by women with hepatic impairment.

A woman who has been using a medication that is a moderate or strong CYP3A4 inhibitor should wait for 2 weeks after the last dose of the CYP3A4 inhibitor before beginning flibanserin. If a woman is initiating a moderate or strong CYP3A4 inhibitor following the use of flibanserin, the CYP3A4 drug therapy should not start until 2 days after the last dose of flibanserin.

Flibanserin can only be prescribed by clinicians who have completed the Addyi Risk Evaluation and Management Strategy (REMS) program and can only be dispensed by pharmacies that have also completed the program. Information on the REMS program and how to participate in the certification process can be found at https://addyi.com/hcp/ or at 1-844-233-9415.

Due to possible adverse events of CNS depression, hypotension, and syncope, flibanserin should not be taken during the day. Bedtime dosing may reduce the risk of injury.

Use with alcohol increases the risk of hypotension and syncope. Women should stop consuming alcohol 2 hours prior to taking flibanserin or skip the dose of flibanserin that evening. Alcohol should not be consumed again until the next morning after an evening dose.

It may take up to 4 weeks for women to see improvement. Treatment should be discontinued after 8 weeks if the woman reports no change.

A missed dose should be skipped. Women should take the next dose at bedtime, but it should not be doubled.

Cost: $$$$$

Fluconazole (Diflucan)

Therapeutic class: Antifungal

Chemical class: Triazole

Indications
Fluconazole is indicated for the treatment of cryptococcal meningitis, esophageal and oropharyngeal candidiasis, and vulvovaginal candidiasis.

Contraindications
Fluconazole is contraindicated with the co-administration of drugs known to prolong the QT interval and known to be metabolized via enzyme CYP3A4. These include astemizole, cisapride, erythromycin, pimozide, and quinidine. Most arrhythmias occur for women with serious, coexisting medical conditions such as advanced heart failure; electrolyte imbalances, including hypokalemia; and structural heart disease.

Co-administration with terfenadine is contraindicated if multiple doses of fluconazole reach or exceed 400 mg.

Fluconazole is contraindicated with known hypersensitivity to the medication and should be used with caution by women who have a hypersensitivity to other azoles.

Mechanism of Action

Fluconazole damages fungal cells by interfering with a cytochrome P-450 enzyme needed to convert lanosterol to ergosterol, an essential part of the fungal cytoplasmic membrane. Decreased ergosterol synthesis causes increased cell permeability and destruction of the cell wall. Fluconazole is primarily fungistatic; however, it may be fungicidal against certain organisms.

Metabolism & Excretion

Hepatic (minimal) and renal

Adverse Reactions

Rare anaphylaxis and exfoliative skin disorders have been reported, but they are unusual with single-dose treatment for vulvovaginal candidiasis.

Side Effects

For women taking 150-mg single-dose fluconazole for vulvovaginal candidiasis, the most common treatment-related side effects are abdominal pain, alterations in taste, diarrhea, headache, and nausea.

Drug–Drug Interactions

Fluconazole is a potent CYP2C9 inhibitor and a moderate CYP3A4 inhibitor. Fluconazole may increase the plasma concentrations of alfentanil, carbamazepine, celecoxib, cyclosporine, fentanyl, glipizide, glyburide, halofantrine, phenytoin, pimozide, rifabutin, tacrolimus, terfenadine, theophylline, tofacitinib, tolbutamide, triazolam, voriconazole, and zidovudine.

QT prolongation may occur, possibly leading to torsades de pointes, if fluconazole is administered with amiodarone, astemizole, cisapride, erythromycin, pimozide, quinidine, or terfenadine.

Fluconazole increases the effect of amitriptyline and nortriptyline and may increase the effects of benzodiazepines and calcium channel blockers.

Fluconazole may increase prothrombin time for women taking coumadin-type anticoagulants, so dose adjustments of the anticoagulant may be necessary.

Other drug interactions are possible. Clinicians should review recent and current medications carefully with women before prescribing fluconazole.

Specific Considerations for Women

Pregnancy

There is a potential for fetal harm if used during pregnancy. Use in pregnancy should be avoided except for women with severe or potentially life-threatening fungal infections when the anticipated benefit outweighs the possible risk to the fetus. Spontaneous abortions and congenital abnormalities have been suggested as potential risks associated with 150 mg of fluconazole as a single or repeated dose in the first trimester of pregnancy.

Distinct congenital anomalies have occurred for infants exposed in utero to high-dose maternal fluconazole (400–800 mg/day) during the first trimester. Effective contraceptive measures should be considered for women of reproductive potential who are being treated with fluconazole 400–800 mg/day and should continue throughout the treatment period and for approximately 1 week after the final dose. If fluconazole is used during pregnancy or if the woman becomes pregnant while taking the drug, she should be informed of the potential hazard to the fetus.

Breastfeeding

Fluconazole is acceptable during breastfeeding. Amounts secreted in human milk are less than the typical neonatal dose.

Adolescent women

Fluconazole can be used by adolescent women.

Elderly women

No differences in safety or effectiveness have been noted between older and younger women. Fluconazole can be used by women over age 65.

Dose: Variable, based on condition being treated

Vulvovaginal candidiasis:
150 mg orally in a single dose

Oropharyngeal candidiasis:
200 mg orally on the first day, followed by 100 mg orally once daily for 2 weeks to decrease the likelihood of relapse.

Esophageal candidiasis:
200 mg orally on the first day, followed by 100 mg orally once daily for a minimum of 3 weeks (or at least 2 weeks after resolution of symptoms). Doses up to 400 mg per day may be used based on the response to therapy.

Systemic candidiasis:
No established dosing regimen; may use doses up to 400 mg orally daily. Consider an infectious disease consult.

Cryptococcal meningitis:
400 mg orally on the first day, followed by 200 to 400 mg orally daily based on response and continued for 10 to 12 weeks after cerebral spinal fluid culture is negative. The dose to suppress relapse for individuals with acquired immune deficiency syndrome is 200 mg orally daily.

How Supplied
Fluconazole is supplied as 50-mg, 100-mg, 150-mg, and 200-mg tablets for oral use.

Prescribing Information
Pregnancy should be avoided during use. Effective contraceptive methods should be used by women who could become pregnant and are being treated with fluconazole 400–800 mg per day. Pregnancy should be avoided throughout the treatment period and for approximately 1 week after the final dose.

Fluconazole should be used with caution by individuals with liver disease, as hepatotoxicity has been reported. Fluconazole should be discontinued if signs of liver disease develop.

Symptoms of vulvovaginal candidiasis should begin to improve within 24 hours but may take several days to completely resolve.

There is potential for drug resistance to fluconazole, and this should be considered if there is no clinical improvement.

Laboratory monitoring for electrolytes, liver function, and renal function is not necessary for single-dose treatment of vulvovaginal candidiasis for otherwise healthy women.

Cost: $

Gabapentin (Gabarone, Gralise, Neurontin)

G

Therapeutic class: Neuropathic pain agent

Chemical class: Anticonvulsant

Indications
Gabapentin is indicated for the treatment of:
1. Postherpetic neuralgia (PHN) among adults
2. Adjunctive therapy for adults with partial onset seizures

   Gabapentin is used off label for the treatment of vulvodynia.

Contraindications
Gabapentin is contraindicated for individuals with known hypersensitivity to pregabalin or any of its components.

Mechanism of Action
The precise mechanisms by which gabapentin produces its analgesic and antiepileptic actions are unknown. Gabapentin interacts with cortical neurons at subunits of calcium channels. Gabapentin increases the synaptic concentration of gamma-aminobutyric acid (GABA), enhances GABA responses at nonsynaptic sites in neuronal tissues, and reduces the release of monoamine neurotransmitters. It may reduce axon excitability in the hippocampus.

Metabolism & Excretion
Minimally metabolized, excreted primarily unchanged in the urine

Adverse Reactions
Potentially serious adverse reactions are possible and include angioedema and multiorgan hypersensitivity reactions, elevated creatine kinase, mood changes, and suicidal thoughts.

Side Effects
Dizziness, fatigue, somnolence, visual disturbances, weight gain

Drug–Drug Interactions
Taking gabapentin with other central nervous system (CNS) depressants such as alcohol, benzodiazepines, and opioids will increase the risk of dizziness, drowsiness, and somnolence.

Antacids containing magnesium and aluminum hydroxide reduce the bioavailability of gabapentin.

Specific Considerations for Women
Pregnancy
There are no well-controlled studies of gabapentin among women who are pregnant, although animal studies have suggested structural abnormalities and growth restriction. The clinical need for the medication should be weighed against possible risks. Healthcare providers are advised to encourage women who are pregnant and taking pregabalin to enroll in the North American Antiepileptic Drug (NAAED) Pregnancy Registry. This can be done by calling 1-888-233-2334 and must be done by women themselves. Registry information can also be found at http://www.aedpregnancyregistry.org/.

Breastfeeding
Limited information suggests that gabapentin is present in low levels in breast milk. Women taking gabapentin may breastfeed, but the infant should be monitored for drowsiness, adequate weight gain, and developmental milestones, especially if the infant is younger and exclusively breastfeeding.

Adolescent women
Gabapentin can be used by adolescent women.

Elderly women
No differences in safety and efficacy have been observed between older and younger individuals. There are no recommended age-related dose reductions other than those based on creatinine clearance.

Dose: Variable, depending on the condition being treated
Postherpetic neuralgia:

> Day 1: 300 mg orally in a single dose
> Day 2: 300 mg orally twice daily
> Day 3: 300 mg orally three times per day

The dose can be titrated as needed for pain relief to 600 mg three times per day (1,800 mg total dose).

Adjunct therapy for partial-onset seizures:
The starting dose is 300 mg orally three times per day. The recommended maintenance dose is 300 mg to 600 mg orally three times per day. Doses can be increased to 2,400 mg per day if needed.

Vulvodynia:
Off label; no formal dosing guidelines exist. In the literature, the doses reported most often for vulvodynia are a starting dose of 300 mg orally daily to a maximum of 1,200 mg orally three times per day (total daily dose of 3,600 mg). The lowest dose to control symptoms should be used.

Dose reductions are required for individuals with renal impairment. Refer to full prescribing information for suggested dose adjustments.

How Supplied
Gabapentin is supplied as 100-mg, 300-mg, 400-mg, 600-mg, and 800-mg capsules or tablets for oral use.

Prescribing Considerations
Gabapentin is not a controlled substance; however, some individuals have reported euphoric effects while taking gabapentin. History of substance abuse should be assessed prior to beginning treatment.

Changes in mood or suicidal thoughts should be reported to a healthcare provider immediately.

Abrupt discontinuation may result in diarrhea, headache, increased seizure activity, insomnia, and nausea. The dose should be gradually reduced over the course of one week.

Alcohol use should be avoided or greatly reduced while taking gabapentin.

Activities that require mental alertness, such as driving, should be avoided until the effects of gabapentin are known.

Individuals with reduced renal function will need lower doses of gabapentin.

Cost: $$

Glipizide (Glucotrol, Glucotrol XL)

Therapeutic class: Antidiabetic

Chemical class: Second-generation sulfonylurea. Other medications in this category include glimepiride and glyburide.

Indications
Glipizide is indicated as an adjunct to diet and exercise to improve glycemic control for adults with type II diabetes mellitus.

Contraindications
Glipizide is contraindicated with known hypersensitivity to the drug. It is also contraindicated for the treatment of type I diabetes mellitus.

Mechanism of Action
Glipizide stimulates insulin secretion from the pancreas.

Metabolism & Excretion
Hepatic and renal

Adverse Reactions

The administration of oral hypoglycemic drugs (including sulfonylureas) has been associated with increased cardiovascular mortality when compared to treatment with diet alone or diet plus insulin.

Hypoglycemia is possible with sulfonylurea medications, including glipizide.

Side Effects

Anemia, diarrhea, dizziness, fatigue, nausea, skin reactions, and vomiting have been reported.

Drug–Drug Interactions

Sulfonylurea medications can cause hemolytic anemia for individuals with glucose 6-phosphate dehydrogenase (G6PD) deficiency.

Some azoles, beta-adrenergic blocking agents, chloramphenicol, coumarins, drugs that are highly protein bound, monoamine oxidase inhibitors, nonsteroidal anti-inflammatory drugs (NSAIDs), probenecid, quinolones, salicylates, and sulfonamides may potentiate the effect of glipizide and result in hypoglycemia.

Calcium channel blocking drugs, corticosteroids, estrogens, isoniazid, nicotinic acid, oral contraceptives, phenothiazines, phenytoin, sympathomimetics, thiazides and other diuretics, and thyroid products may cause hyperglycemia.

Specific Considerations for Women

Pregnancy

There are no adequate and well-controlled studies of glipizide use by women who are pregnant. According to the American Diabetes Association (ADA) and the American College of Obstetricians and Gynecologists (ACOG), insulin should be considered the first-line drug if pharmacologic control of blood sugar is necessary during pregnancy. Oral agents can be considered if women are unable or unwilling to inject insulin or if they can't afford insulin. Metformin may be an alternative oral medication.

Breastfeeding
There are limited data on glipizide and breastfeeding, although levels in breast milk appear to be low. Women who are breastfeeding and taking glucose-lowering medications should monitor their infants for signs of hypoglycemia. Other drugs to consider during breastfeeding include glyburide, insulin, and metformin.

Adolescent women
Safety and efficacy have not been established for individuals under age 18.

Elderly women
No differences in safety or effectiveness have been noted between older and younger women.

Individuals who are older may be at increased risk of hypoglycemia. Consider initiating treatment at the lowest dosing range.

Dose
The recommended starting dose of glipizide is 5 mg, given orally prior to breakfast. The maximum daily dose is 40 mg, and no more than 15 mg should be taken at any one time. Divided doses should be taken prior to meals. Dose adjustments should occur in 2.5-mg or 5-mg amounts.

The recommended starting dose of glipizide XL is 5 mg once daily, given orally prior to breakfast. The maximum daily dose is 20 mg once daily.

How Supplied
Glipizide is supplied as 5-mg and 10-mg tablets for oral use.

Glipizide XL is supplied as 2.5-mg, 5-mg, and 10-mg tablets for oral use.

Prescribing Considerations
Glipizide should be taken 30 minutes prior to meals.

Periodic monitoring of blood glucose through glycosylated hemoglobin or daily measurements is prudent and will help guide dose changes.

Glipizide should always be used in conjunction with dietary and lifestyle changes to reduce hyperglycemia.

Cost: $$

Hydrochlorothiazide (HydroDIURIL, Microzide, and others)

Therapeutic class: Antihypertensive, diuretic

Chemical class: Thiazide diuretic

Indications
Hydrochlorothiazide (HCTZ) is indicated for the management of hypertension, either alone or with other antihypertensives.

Contraindications
HCTZ is contraindicated with hypersensitivity to the drug or other sulfonamide drugs. HCTZ should not be used by individuals with anuria.

Diuretics reduce the renal clearance of lithium and may cause lithium toxicity. Concurrent use should be avoided.

Mechanism of Action
HCTZ blocks the reabsorption of sodium and chloride ions and increases the quantity of sodium through the distal tubule and the volume of water excreted. Antihypertensive effects of thiazides occur from a reduction in blood volume and cardiac output.

Metabolism & Excretion
No significant metabolism; excreted renally

Adverse Reactions
HCTZ may cause acute closed-angle glaucoma, azotemia, and myopia for individuals with renal failure.

Hypercalcemia, hyperuricemia, and hypokalemia may occur.

Side Effects
Dizziness, hypotension, skin rashes, vertigo, and weakness have occurred with doses of HCTZ over 25 mg.

Drug–Drug Interactions
Sedatives such as alcohol, barbiturates, and opioids may increase the risk for orthostatic hypotension.

Other antihypertensives will potentiate the effect of HCTZ.

Concurrent use of HCTZ with corticosteroids may increase electrolyte depletion.

When HCTZ is given with antidiabetic agents, the dose of the antidiabetic drug may have to be adjusted.

Specific Considerations for Women

Pregnancy

HCTZ is generally not recommended during pregnancy, although there is no indication that exposure to HCTZ causes fetal harm. Diuretics are not used to treat pregnancy-associated edema. Labetalol is commonly used to treat hypertension in pregnancy.

Breastfeeding

HCTZ is excreted in breast milk. HCTZ in doses of 50 mg or less per day are acceptable during breastfeeding. Increased diuresis from large doses will decrease the quantity of breast milk.

Adolescent women

HCTZ may be used by adolescents.

Elderly women

A greater blood pressure reduction and an increase in side effects may be observed among individuals over 65 years of age. HCTZ should be initiated at the lowest available dose of 12.5 mg and doses titrated by no more than 12.5 mg at one time.

Dose

The initial dose is 12.5 mg orally once daily. The dose may be increased up to 50 mg daily in a single dose or 2 divided doses.

How Supplied

HCTZ is supplied as 12.5-mg, 25-mg, and 50-mg tablets or capsules for oral use.

Prescribing Considerations

Taking HCTZ in the morning will reduce the chance of increased urination at night.

Electrolytes should be assessed at least yearly for individuals taking HCTZ.

Cost: $

Hydroxyzine (Vistaril)

Therapeutic class: Antiemetic, antipruritic, anxiolytic, sedative

Chemical class: First-generation histamine H1 antagonist

Indications
Hydroxyzine is indicated for symptomatic relief of anxiety and tension in organic disease states in which anxiety is manifested. It is also indicated for allergic conditions such as atopic and contact dermatoses and chronic urticaria, and in histamine-mediated pruritus.

Contraindications
Hydroxyzine is contraindicated during early pregnancy due to evidence of fetal abnormalities in animal models. It is also contraindicated with a known allergy or hypersensitivity to the medication.

Mechanism of Action
Hydroxyzine is a direct competitor of histamine for binding at cellular receptor sites and produces antianxiety and sedative effects through suppression of activity at subcortical levels.

Metabolism & Excretion
Hepatic and renal

Adverse Reactions
No major adverse reactions have been noted.

Side Effects
Hydroxyzine may cause allergic reactions, drowsiness, dry mouth, and sedation.

Drug–Drug Interactions
Concomitant use with other central nervous system (CNS) depressants such as alcohol, barbiturates, or opioids will potentiate CNS depression and sedation.

Use with other anticholinergic agents will increase anticholinergic effects.

Specific Considerations for Women
Pregnancy
Hydroxyzine is contraindicated during early pregnancy due to evidence of fetal abnormalities in animal models.

Breastfeeding
Small and occasional doses of hydroxyzine are not expected to cause adverse effects for infants who are breastfeeding. Larger doses for a prolonged time may cause infant drowsiness or a decreased milk supply. Cetirizine may be considered as an alternative treatment for pruritus.

Adolescent women
Hydroxyzine is approved for use by children and may be used by adolescent women.

Elderly women
No differences in safety or effectiveness have been noted between older and younger women. Individuals who are older may experience more sedating effects compared with those who are younger.

Dose
Anxiety:
50 mg or 100 mg orally four times per day

Pruritus:
25 mg orally three to four times per day

How Supplied
Hydroxyzine is available as 10-mg, 25-mg, 50-mg, and 100-mg tablets for oral use and 25-mg, 50-mg, and 100-mg capsules for oral use.

Prescribing Considerations

Sedation may occur, especially at higher doses. Activities that require mental alertness should be avoided until individuals know how they react to hydroxyzine.

Alcohol and other sedatives should be avoided with use of hydroxyzine.

Vaginal dryness is possible due to the antihistamine effects of the medication.

Cost: $

Imiquimod cream, 5% (Aldara)

Therapeutic class: Keratolytic

Chemical class: Immune response modifier

Indications

Imiquimod cream is indicated for the treatment of external genital warts (EGWs) for individuals 12 years of age or older.

Also approved for treatment of nonhyperkeratotic, nonhypertrophic actinic keratoses on the face or scalp of adults and primary superficial basal cell carcinoma.

This book focuses on imiquimod cream for the treatment of EGWs.

Contraindications

None known

Mechanism of Action

The mechanism of action of imiquimod cream in the treatment of EGWs is unknown. Imiquimod has no direct antiviral activity but appears to induce mRNA encoding cytokines, including interferon-α, at the treatment site. How this relates to clearance of EGWs is unclear.

Metabolism & Excretion

Not applicable

Adverse Reactions
Significant vulvar edema leading to urinary retention has been reported.

Side Effects
Local inflammatory skin reactions are common and an expected part of treatment with imiquimod cream. These include burning, edema, erythema, excoriation, pain, pruritus, and skin weeping. Such reactions can occur within a few days of application. Treatment interruption may be necessary in cases of significant skin reactions. Influenza-like symptoms, including chills, fever, and myalgias, may precede local inflammatory reactions.

Drug–Drug Interactions
There are no known clinically significant drug–drug interactions.

Specific Considerations for Women
Pregnancy
There are no well-controlled studies of imiquimod cream use among women who are pregnant. EGWs need not be removed during pregnancy, and the use of imiquimod cream can be delayed until after delivery. Women who are pregnant and have large or friable EGWs should speak with their healthcare provider about all available options for condyloma removal.

Breastfeeding
It is not known if imiquimod is excreted into breast milk. However, only minimal amounts of the medication are absorbed systemically from topical application, making it unlikely that high concentrations would be present in breast milk.

Adolescent women
Imiquimod cream can be used by women beginning at age 12.

Elderly women
Imiquimod cream has been evaluated on women older than age 65. No clinically significant differences were noted between younger and older women.

Dose
For the treatment of EGWs, imiquimod cream is applied in a thin layer directly to the EGWs, 3 times per week (application schedule examples include Monday, Wednesday, Friday or Tuesday, Thursday, Saturday). Applications should continue until clearance or up to a maximum of 16 weeks. The cream is applied at bedtime and left on the skin for 6 to 10 hours, then washed off.

How Supplied
Imiquimod cream 5% is supplied in single-use packets (24 per box), each of which contains 250 mg of the cream, equivalent to 12.5 mg of imiquimod.

Prescribing Considerations
Exposure to sunlight, including artificial light from tanning beds, should be avoided or minimized while using imiquimod cream due to the increased potential for sunburn.

Sexual activity should be avoided while imiquimod cream is on the skin.

Imiquimod cream may weaken latex condoms and diaphragms; the cream should not come in contact with these products.

Imiquimod cream is for external use only and should not be used rectally, at the urethral meatus, or in the vagina. If imiquimod cream is used by women during their menstrual cycle, it should be applied after a tampon or menstrual cup is inserted to avoid possibly introducing the cream into the vagina.

The treatment area should not be occluded or bandaged.

New EGWs may develop during treatment and it is unknown if removal of EGWs reduces transmission.

Significant local skin reactions should be evaluated by a healthcare provider.

Vaccination with the 9-valent human papilloma virus vaccine should be considered as a routine vaccine.

Cost: $$$$$

Ivermectin (Stromectol)

Therapeutic class: Anthelmintic

Chemical class: Pediculicide

Indications
Ivermectin is indicated for the treatment of intestinal strongyloidiasis and onchocerciasis. It is frequently used off-label for the treatment of scabies and lice.

Contraindications
Ivermectin is contraindicated for individuals with a known allergy or hypersensitivity to the medication.

Mechanism of Action
Ivermectin binds selectively to glutamate-gated chloride ion channels that occur in invertebrate nerve and muscle cells. This leads to an increase in the permeability of the cell membrane to chloride ions, resulting in paralysis and death of the parasite.

Metabolism & Excretion
Hepatic and gastrointestinal (fecal)

Adverse Reactions
Microfilaricidal drugs, and drugs such as ivermectin, may cause potentially serious cutaneous or systemic reactions (Mazzotti reaction) and ophthalmological reactions for individuals with onchocerciasis. These reactions are probably due to allergic and inflammatory responses to the death of microfilariae.

Side Effects
Diarrhea, dizziness, nausea, pruritis, and rash.

Drug–Drug Interactions
An increased international normalized ratio (INR) may occur if ivermectin is taken with warfarin.

Specific Considerations for Women

Pregnancy

There are no well-controlled studies of ivermectin use by women who are pregnant. Topical agents should be considered if treatment for scabies or lice is needed during pregnancy.

Breastfeeding

Oral ivermectin is excreted in breast milk, but limited data indicate that levels are low. Amounts ingested by the infant are small and would not be expected to cause any adverse effects. However, a topical agent for scabies or lice should be considered as an alternate treatment during breastfeeding.

Adolescent women

Ivermectin can be used by adolescent women.

Elderly women

No differences in safety or effectiveness have been noted between older and younger women.

Dose: Variable, depending on condition being treated

Head lice:

A single oral dose designed to provide approximately 200 mcg of ivermectin per kg of body weight. A second dose may be required if visible nits are present.

Onchocerciasis:

A single oral dose designed to provide approximately 150 mcg of ivermectin per kg of body weight.

Scabies: Two oral doses, approximately one week apart, each designed to provide approximately 200 mcg of ivermectin per kg of body weight.

Crusted scabies: Depending on severity, three doses (approximately days 1, 2, and 8), five doses (approximately days 1, 2, 8, 9, and 15), or seven doses (approximately days 1, 2, 8, 9, 15, 22, and 29), each designed to provide approximately 200 mcg of ivermectin per kg of body weight. Oral ivermectin should also be used with a topical agent for crusted scabies.

Strongyloidiasis:
A single oral dose designed to provide approximately 200 mcg of ivermectin per kg of body weight.

How Supplied
Ivermectin is supplied as 3-mg tablets for oral use.

Prescribing Considerations
Ivermectin should be taken on an empty stomach with water when treating worm infestations, but taking the medication with food may increase the bioavailability when treating scabies.

Ivermectin is not a first-line treatment for scabies, but it may be considered if topical agents have failed.

Use of oral ivermectin for scabies and lice is off label.

Cost: $–$$

Labetalol hydrochloride (Nomodyne, Trandate)

Therapeutic class: Antihypertensive

Chemical class: Beta-blocker. Other drugs in this category include atenolol, carvedilol, metoprolol, and propranolol.

Indications
Labetalol is indicated for the management of hypertension. Labetalol may be used alone or in combination with other antihypertensive agents, especially thiazide and loop diuretics.

Contraindications
Beta-blockers, including labetalol (even those with cardioselectivity), should not be used by individuals with a history of obstructive airway disease, including asthma.

Labetalol is also contraindicated with cardiogenic shock, hypersensitivity to the medication, greater-than-first-degree heart block, overt cardiac failure, severe bradycardia, and other conditions associated with significant hypotension.

Mechanism of Action
Labetalol blocks beta 1-receptors in the heart, beta 2-receptors in bronchial and vascular smooth muscle, and alpha 1-receptors in vascular smooth muscle. This leads to vasodilation and decreased total peripheral resistance, which results in decreased blood pressure without a substantial decrease in cardiac output, resting heart rate, or stroke volume.

Metabolism & Elimination
Hepatic and renal

Adverse Reactions
Serious adverse reactions include bronchospasm, cardiac failure, hepatic injury, ischemic heart disease with abrupt discontinuation, and paradoxical hypertensive responses for individuals with pheochromocytoma. Additionally, the metabolism of labetalol may be reduced in the presence of impaired hepatic function.

Side Effects
Dizziness, fatigue, nausea

Drug–Drug Interactions
Beta-blockers reduce the release of insulin in response to hyperglycemia, and the dose of antidiabetic drugs may have to be adjusted.

Cimetidine has been associated with an increased bioavailability of labetalol.

Beta-blockers and digitalis slow atrioventricular conduction and decrease heart rate. Concomitant use can increase the risk of bradycardia.

Specific Considerations for Women
Pregnancy
Labetalol is considered a first-line drug to treat hypertension during pregnancy, including management of chronic hypertension and hypertensive emergencies. There is no evidence of fetal harm.

Breastfeeding
Labetalol is excreted in breast milk in low amounts. Labetalol is acceptable during breastfeeding if pharmacologic treatment of hypertension is necessary.

Adolescent women
Data on use of labetalol by adolescents is limited, but the drug may be used to treat hypertension in this population.

Elderly women
Individuals over age 60 may experience increased episodes of dizziness, lightheadedness, and orthostatic hypotension, which could increase the risk for falls. The lowest starting dose, and slow titration and taper, should be considered.

Dose
The recommended initial dose is 100 mg orally twice daily, used alone or with a diuretic. After 2 or 3 days, the dose may be titrated in increments of 100 mg twice daily. Increases may occur every 2 or 3 days. The usual maintenance dose of labetalol ranges from 200 mg to 400 mg orally twice daily.

How Supplied
Labetalol is supplied as 100-mg and 200-mg tablets for oral use.

Prescribing Considerations
Blood pressure should be evaluated in the office setting prior to dose titration.

When discontinuing labetalol after prolonged administration, especially for individuals with ischemic heart disease, the dose should be gradually reduced over a period of 1 to 2 weeks.

Other beta-blockers are available that may have a different dosing schedule and cost. Choice of medication should be individualized to the specific needs of each woman.

Cost: $–$$

Ledipasvir/Sofosbuvir (Harvoni)

Therapeutic class: Direct-acting antiviral (DAA)

Chemical class: Hepatitis C virus (HCV) NS5A inhibitor/HCV nucleotide analog NS5B polymerase inhibitor

Indications
Ledipasvir/sofosbuvir is indicated in the treatment of HCV for:

1. Adults with genotype 1, 4, 5, or 6 infection without cirrhosis or with compensated cirrhosis
2. Adults with genotype 1 infection with decompensated cirrhosis, in combination with ribavirin
3. Adults with genotype 1 or 4 infection who are liver transplant recipients without cirrhosis or with compensated cirrhosis, in combination with ribavirin
4. Children 12 years of age and older or weighing at least 35 kg (77 lb) with genotype 1, 4, 5, or 6 without cirrhosis or with compensated cirrhosis

Contraindications
Co-administration of ledipasvir/sofosbuvir with P-gp inducers such as rifampin and St. John's wort may significantly decrease ledipasvir and sofosbuvir plasma concentrations and may lead to a reduced therapeutic effect. The use of ledipasvir/sofosbuvir with P-gp inducers is not recommended.

Co-administration of amiodarone with ledipasvir/sofosbuvir is not recommended due to the possibility of serious and symptomatic bradycardia.

Mechanism of Action
Ledipasvir is an inhibitor of the HCV NS5A protein, and sofosbuvir is an inhibitor of the HCV NS5B RNA-dependent RNA polymerase, both of which are required for viral replication.

Metabolism & Elimination
Hepatic and renal

Adverse Reactions
Ledipasvir/sofosbuvir may cause a reactivation of hepatitis B virus (HBV) for individuals coinfected with HBV and HCV.

Side Effects
Asthenia, diarrhea, fatigue, headache, nausea

Drug–Drug Interactions
Acid-reducing agents, anticonvulsants, antimycobacterials, St. John's wort, and tipranavir/ritonavir may all reduce the concentration of ledipasvir/sofosbuvir.

Ledipasvir/sofosbuvir may increase the concentrations of atorvastatin, digoxin, rosuvastatin, and tenofovir.

There are many potential drug–drug interactions with ledipasvir/sofosbuvir in addition to the ones listed. A careful history, review of current medications, and review of the full drug information should be done prior to prescribing.

Specific Considerations for Women
Pregnancy
Based on animal data and limited human data, ledipasvir/sofosbuvir does not appear to adversely affect the fetus. However, no DAA therapy has been approved to treat HCV during pregnancy. Currently it is recommended that HCV treatment be deferred until after delivery. Decisions regarding use of DAAs during pregnancy should be made on an individual basis, weighing risks of untreated HCV against possible unknown fetal risks.

Breastfeeding
Treatment with ledipasvir/sofosbuvir for HCV is not a reason to discontinue breastfeeding. Among all DAAs, both ledipasvir and sofosbuvir have a favorable profile for lactation.

Adolescent women
Ledipasvir/sofosbuvir is approved for treatment of HCV for adolescent women.

Elderly women

No overall differences in safety or effectiveness have been observed between older and younger individuals.

Dose

Ledipasvir/sofosbuvir is taken as one tablet orally once per day for a minimum of 12 weeks, with or without ribavirin. See full prescribing information for when to consider adding ribavirin.

How Supplied

Each fixed-dose tablet for oral use contains 90 mg ledipasvir and 400 mg sofosbuvir.

Prescribing Considerations

Ledipasvir/sofosbuvir has a **black box warning** for the possibility of HBV reactivation for individuals who are coinfected with HBV and HCV.

All individuals should be tested for HBV prior to initiating treatment with ledipasvir/sofosbuvir.

If ledipasvir/sofosbuvir is administered with ribavirin, the warnings and precautions for ribavirin, including the need to avoid pregnancy, apply to this combination regimen.

Due to multiple drug–drug interactions, a careful medication history should be taken prior to beginning treatment with ledipasvir/sofosbuvir.

Other DAAs are available for the treatment of HCV that may have a different cost and side effect profile. Choice of medication should be individualized to the specific needs of each woman.

Cost: $$$$$

Letrozole (Femara)

Therapeutic class: Antiestrogen

Chemical class: Aromatase inhibitor

Indications
Letrozole is indicated for:

1. Adjuvant treatment for women who are postmenopausal with hormone receptor positive early breast cancer
2. Extended adjuvant treatment for women who are postmenopausal with early breast cancer who have received prior standard adjuvant tamoxifen therapy
3. First- and second-line treatment for women who are postmenopausal with hormone receptor positive or unknown advanced breast cancer

Contraindications
Letrozole is contraindicated during pregnancy.

Mechanism of Action
Letrozole is an inhibitor of the aromatase enzyme system and blocks the conversion of androgens to estrogens. The growth of some cancers of the breast is stimulated or maintained by estrogens. Interventions to decrease or block estrogen can lead to decreased tumor mass or delayed progression of tumor growth for some women.

Metabolism & Elimination
Hepatic and renal

Adverse Reactions
Potential adverse effects include bone and joint pain, decreased bone mineral density (BMD), hypercholesterolemia, and somnolence.

Side Effects
Dizziness, fatigue, hot flashes/flushes, menstrual irregularities, night sweats, weight changes

Drug–Drug Interactions
Co-administration of letrozole and tamoxifen decreases serum letrozole levels.

Specific Considerations for Women

Pregnancy

Letrozole may cause fetal harm and is contraindicated during pregnancy. Letrozole has been associated with spontaneous abortions and birth defects. Letrozole is indicated for women who are postmenopausal.

Breastfeeding

There are no available data on the use of letrozole during lactation. Letrozole has antiestrogen properties and may interfere with milk quality and quantity. Per drug labeling, women should not breastfeed while taking letrozole and for 3 weeks after finishing treatment.

Adolescent women

Conditions for which letrozole are indicated generally do not occur during adolescence. The safety and efficacy of letrozole have not been established for women under age 18, and the medication is currently approved for use only by women who are postmenopausal.

Elderly women

No differences in safety or effectiveness have been noted between older and younger women who are postmenopausal.

Dose

The recommended dose is 2.5 mg orally every day. Individuals with severe hepatic impairment or cirrhosis should reduce the dose to 2.5 mg orally every other day.

How Supplied

Letrozole is supplied as a 2.5-mg tablet for oral use.

Prescribing Considerations

Effective contraception is required if letrozole is used during the perimenopausal period.

Women taking letrozole should have a lipid profile done at least yearly during treatment.

Consideration should be given to monitoring BMD during treatment with letrozole, but no information exists to guide frequency of BMD assessments.

Calcium and vitamin D supplementation can be considered if dietary intake is inadequate.

Cost: $$

Leuprolide acetate depot injection (Lupron)

Therapeutic class: Hormone

Chemical class: Synthetic analogue of gonadotropin releasing hormone (GnRH)

Indications
Leuprolide (3.75 mg) is indicated for the management of endometriosis, including pain and reduction of endometriotic lesions. Additionally, this dose, when combined with iron therapy, is indicated for preoperative hematologic improvement of anemia caused by uterine fibroids.

Leuprolide (11.25 mg) is indicated for the management of endometriosis, including pain and reduction of endometriotic lesions.

Contraindications
Leuprolide is contraindicated for women with known hypersensitivity to GnRH or any other component of the medication.

Leuprolide should not be used by women who are pregnant, breastfeeding, or have undiagnosed vaginal bleeding.

Mechanism of Action
Leuprolide acetate is a long-acting GnRH analogue. After injection, there is an initial rise in sex steroids followed by prolonged suppression of pituitary gonadotropins and decreased secretion of gonadal steroids. Tissues and functions that depend on gonadal steroids for their maintenance become quiescent.

Metabolism & Elimination
Hepatic and renal

Adverse Reactions
The hypoestrogenic state caused by leuprolide results in the loss of bone mineral density (BMD). Add-back norethindrone acetate may reduce bone loss.

Anaphylactic, asthmatic, and convulsive reactions have occurred.

A flair of endometriosis symptoms may occur during the first few days after initial treatment due to the rise in sex steroids.

Depression may occur or worsen during treatment with leuprolide.

Side Effects
Decreased libido, depression, dizziness, emotional lability, headache, hot flashes/flushes, nausea, pain at injection site, sweating, vaginitis, vomiting, weight gain

Drug–Drug Interactions
There are no known clinically significant drug–drug interactions.

Specific Considerations for Women
Pregnancy

Leuprolide may cause fetal harm and should not be used by women who are pregnant. Major fetal anomalies have been noted in animal studies. Pregnancy should be excluded prior to injection and nonhormonal contraception used during treatment.

Breastfeeding

There is no information on leuprolide and breastfeeding. The effects on breast milk quality and quantity and adverse effects for the infant are unknown. Leuprolide should not be used during lactation.

Adolescent women

The safety and efficacy of leuprolide have not been established in the treatment of fibroids and endometriosis for women under age 18.

Elderly women

Leuprolide is not indicated for women who are postmenopausal.

Dose

Leuprolide is given as an intramuscular (IM) injection by a healthcare provider of 3.75 mg every month for 3 months or 11.25 mg every 3 months. Total length of treatment is 6 months. Leuprolide may be given alone or with add-back norethindrone acetate 5 mg daily.

How Supplied

Leuprolide acetate is available as a suspension for IM injection in 3.75-mg (one-month) and 11.25-mg (three-month) doses.

Prescribing Considerations

A course of treatment is 6 months. If symptoms reoccur, retreatment for an additional 6 months can be considered, but only with add-back norethindrone acetate 5 mg daily. BMD should be assessed prior to extending treatment beyond the initial 6 months.

Leuprolide is also available as a combination pack containing leuprolide injection and 30 tablets of norethindrone acetate 5 mg. Providers should take care to prescribe the correct formulation that is appropriate for individual women.

If used preoperatively prior to fibroid surgery, duration of treatment is limited to 3 months. Symptoms associated with fibroids will return once treatment is discontinued.

For women with major risk factors for decreased BMD, such as chronic alcohol or tobacco use, chronic use of drugs that decrease BMD, or strong family history of osteoporosis, use of leuprolide will present an additional risk.

Normal function of the pituitary-gonadal system is expected within 3 months after discontinuation of treatment.

Due to the potential for fetal harm, pregnancy should be excluded prior to the initiation of treatment.

Although ovulation is often suppressed during treatment, leuprolide is not a contraceptive method. Women who are sexually active should use a nonhormonal method of contraception during treatment.

Cost: $$$$$

Levonorgestrel emergency contraception (Plan B One-Step and numerous generic brands)

Therapeutic class: Hormone

Chemical class: Progesterone congeners

Indications
Levonorgestrel for emergency contraception is indicated for the prevention of pregnancy after contraceptive failure or unprotected intercourse.

Contraindications
In the United States, package labeling for levonorgestrel for emergency contraception states that it is contraindicated in pregnancy. This is not because the medication is harmful but because the medication provides no therapeutic benefit.

Mechanism of Action
Levonorgestrel for emergency contraception works by impairing ovulation and luteal function. Earlier research suggested that levonorgestrel may alter tubal transport of sperm and/or egg and/or alter the endometrium. However, more recent research suggests that disrupted ovulation is the primary mechanism of action.

Metabolism & Excretion
Hepatic and renal

Adverse Reactions
An increase in ectopic pregnancies has been noted among women who become pregnant while taking progesterone-only contraception. How this relates to a single dose of levonorgestrel for emergency contraception is unknown. Consider the possibility of ectopic pregnancy after use of levonorgestrel for emergency contraception if the woman has a positive pregnancy test, lower abdominal pain, or any other symptoms of an ectopic pregnancy.

Side Effects
The medication is generally well tolerated. Women have reported changes in menses, fatigue, headache, lower abdominal pain, and nausea.

Drug–Drug Interactions
Drugs or herbal products that induce enzymes, including CYP3A4, that metabolize progestins may decrease the plasma concentrations of levonorgestrel and therefore decrease effectiveness. These include barbiturates, bosentan, carbamazepine, felbamate, griseofulvin, oxcarbazepine, phenytoin, rifampin, St. John's wort, and topiramate.

Specific Considerations for Women
Pregnancy
Levonorgestrel for emergency contraception is indicated for the prevention of pregnancy and therefore not indicated for use by pregnant women. However, there are no adverse effects on the fetus if levonorgestrel is taken prior to the diagnosis of pregnancy. Levonorgestrel 1.5 mg is not an abortifacient and will not terminate an existing pregnancy.

Breastfeeding
Small amounts of progestins pass into the breast milk of women who are breastfeeding. No adverse effects have been found on milk quality, quantity, or infant growth and development. Woman who require emergency contraception while breastfeeding may take levonorgestrel for this indication.

Adolescent women
Levonorgestrel for emergency contraception can be used by adolescent women.

Elderly women
This medication is not intended for use by women who are postmenopausal as they are not at risk for pregnancy.

Dose
A single dose (1.5-mg tablet) should be taken as soon as possible after unprotected intercourse or contraceptive failure, but no longer than 120 hours (5 days) thereafter.

How Supplied
Levonorgestrel for emergency contraception is supplied as a single tablet containing 1.5 mg of levonorgestrel.

Prescribing Considerations
Levonorgestrel 1.5 mg as emergency contraception is available in U.S. pharmacies, without a prescription, to anyone, regardless of age. Because many U.S. health insurance plans only cover prescription medications, this will be an out-of-pocket cost for most women.

Levonorgestrel for emergency contraception should be taken within 72 hours of unprotected intercourse, according to package labeling. This can be extended to 120 hours (5 days), but effectiveness decreases with time.

Obesity may decrease the bioavailability of levonorgestrel for emergency contraception. In some research studies, efficacy to prevent pregnancy was significantly reduced among women whose body mass index (BMI) was in the overweight or obese categories. This is an area of ongoing research. Women seeking emergency contraception should be aware of all options.

Levonorgestrel for emergency contraception will not prevent HIV or sexually transmitted infections (STIs).

Menstrual cycle changes may occur, and menses could be early or delayed. If menses don't occur within 3 weeks of taking emergency contraception, the woman should take a pregnancy test.

Levonorgestrel as emergency contraception is less effective than regular contraceptive methods, although repeated use is not harmful. Women should be advised to consider a regular method of contraception that provides a higher level of efficacy.

Cost: $$–$$$

Levothyroxine (Levothroid, Levoxyl, Synthroid, Unithroid)

Therapeutic class: Thyroid hormone replacement

Chemical class: Thyroxine

Indications

Levothyroxine is indicated for:

1. Replacement or supplement for congenital or acquired hypothyroidism
2. Treatment or prevention of euthyroid goiters, including thyroid nodules, thyroiditis, and multinodular goiter

Contraindications

Levothyroxine is contraindicated for individuals with:

1. Untreated subclinical or overt thyrotoxicosis of any etiology
2. Acute myocardial infarction
3. Uncorrected adrenal insufficiency

Mechanism of Action

Levothyroxine exhibits all the actions of endogenous thyroid hormone. Thyroid hormones affect tissue growth and maturation and increase energy expenditure. This is accomplished through control of DNA transcription and protein synthesis.

Metabolism & Excretion

Hepatic and renal

Adverse Reactions

For women, long-term levothyroxine therapy has been associated with decreased bone mineral density (BMD), especially among women who are postmenopausal and receiving large doses.

Levothyroxine should be used with caution by women with underlying cardiac disease as the dose may have to be reduced. Arrhythmias and angina are possible.

Hypersensitivity reactions, including pruritus, rash, and urticaria, have occurred.

Side Effects

Diarrhea, fatigue, flushing, hair loss, headache, heat intolerance, irritability, menstrual irregularities, nausea, vomiting, and weight loss have been reported.

Drug–Drug Interactions

There are many potential drug interactions with levothyroxine. Highlights are provided, but full prescribing information should be consulted.

Drugs that may result in hypothyroidism: aminoglutethimide, amiodarone, antacids, bile acid sequestrants, calcium carbonate, carbamazepine, ferrous sulfate, hydantoins, iodine, lithium, methimazole, orlistat, phenobarbital, propylthiouracil (PTU), rifampin, sucralfate, sulfonamides, and tolbutamide.

Thyroid hormones appear to increase the catabolism of vitamin K-dependent clotting factors and therefore increase the anticoagulant activity of oral anticoagulants.

Concurrent use of antidepressants, including selective serotonin reuptake inhibitors (SSRIs), tetracyclics, and tricyclics, with levothyroxine may increase the therapeutic and toxic effects of both drugs.

Concomitant use of levothyroxine and antidiabetic or insulin agents may result in increased antidiabetic agent or insulin requirements.

Serum digitalis levels may be reduced in hyperthyroidism or when the individual who has hypothyroidism is converted to the euthyroid state.

Concomitant use of levothyroxine and ketamine may result in marked hypertension and tachycardia.

Specific Considerations for Women

Pregnancy

Fetal harm has not been reported. Levothyroxine requirements may be increased during pregnancy. Hypothyroidism during pregnancy has been associated with a higher rate of complications, including pre-eclampsia, preterm birth, spontaneous abortion, and stillbirth. Maternal hypothyroidism may have an adverse effect on fetal and childhood growth and development. Women who are pregnant and taking levothyroxine should have their thyroid stimulating hormone (TSH) level measured during each trimester. The dose of levothyroxine may have to be adjusted and a serum TSH level should be obtained at 6 to 8 weeks postpartum.

Breastfeeding
Levothyroxine is excreted in breast milk in small amounts. Normal levels are required to maintain adequate lactation. Women may breastfeed while taking levothyroxine.

Adolescent women
Safety and efficacy of levothyroxine have been established for adolescent women. See dosing guidelines.

Elderly women
Dose reductions are often needed for women over age 50. See dosing guidelines.

Dose
Dosing guidelines are variable and depend on many factors, including age, other medications, underlying medical condition, weight, and whether the woman is pregnant.

General guidelines for oral doses:

Healthy women less than age 50:
Average full replacement dose is approximately 1.7 mcg/kg/day (100–125 mcg/day for a 70-kg [154-lb] adult).

Women over age 50 or younger women with cardiac disease:
Initial starting dose of 25–50 mcg/day is recommended; increase dose as needed at 6- to 8-week intervals.

Women with severe hypothyroidism:
Initial starting dose is 12.5–25 mcg/day; may be increased by 25 mcg/day every 2 to 4 weeks until the TSH is normal.

Adolescent women over age 12:
2–3 mcg/kg/day

Adolescent women with growth and puberty complete:
1.7 mcg/kg/day

How Supplied
Levothyroxine is available as 25-mcg, 50-mcg, 75-mcg, 88-mcg, 100-mcg, 112-mcg, 125-mcg, 137-mcg, 150-mcg, 175-mcg, 200-mcg, and 300-mcg tablets for oral use.

Prescribing Considerations
Levothyroxine has a **black box warning** stating that thyroid hormones, including levothyroxine, should not be used for weight loss or obesity treatment. Large doses may produce life-threatening toxicity.

Levothyroxine has a long half-life, and the peak therapeutic effect may not be attained for 4 to 6 weeks.

Levothyroxine has a narrow therapeutic window. Careful titration is necessary.

Dose adjustments typically occur in 12.5- to 25-mcg increments, based on TSH levels.

Levothyroxine should be taken in the morning on an empty stomach. Women should wait 30 minutes after taking the medication before eating.

There are many drug–drug interactions with levothyroxine. The full prescribing information of each medication should be consulted if a woman is taking levothyroxine and needs additional medication.

Cost: $

Linaclotide (Linzess)

Therapeutic class: Anti-irritable bowel agent

Chemical class: Guanylate cyclase-C agonist

Indications
Linaclotide is indicated for the treatment of adults with idiopathic chronic constipation and irritable bowel syndrome with constipation (IBS-C).

Contraindications
Linaclotide is contraindicated for individuals under age 18 and for individuals with a known or suspected mechanical bowel obstruction.

Mechanism of Action
Linaclotide functions as a guanylate cyclase-C (GC-C) agonist, binds to GC-C, and acts locally on the luminal surface of the intestinal epithelium. Concentrations of cyclic guanosine monophosphate (cGMP) are increased, which stimulates secretion of chloride and bicarbonate into the intestinal lumen, resulting in increased intestinal fluid and accelerated transit.

Metabolism & Excretion
Gastrointestinal

Adverse Reactions
Dehydration, possibly fatal, can occur if linaclotide is taken by children. See contraindications.

Side Effects
Abdominal pain, bloating, diarrhea, flatulence

Drug–Drug Interactions
There are no known clinically significant drug–drug interactions.

Specific Considerations for Women
Pregnancy
Linaclotide and its active metabolite are negligibly absorbed systemically, and maternal use is not expected to result in exposure to the fetus. Data are lacking on the use of linaclotide during pregnancy, and therefore definitive information on any drug-associated risk for major birth defects and pregnancy loss is not available. In animal studies, no effects on embryo-fetal development were observed. Until more data are available, constipation during pregnancy should be managed with other methods.

Breastfeeding
No lactation studies have been conducted and there is no information on the presence of linaclotide in human milk, or its effects on milk production

or infants who are breastfeeding. Linaclotide and its active metabolite are negligibly absorbed systemically following oral administration, but it is unknown whether the negligible systemic absorption of linaclotide will affect exposure for breastfeeding infants. Until more data are available, constipation during lactation should be managed with other methods.

Adolescent women
Linaclotide is contraindicated for individuals under age 18.

Elderly women
No differences in safety or effectiveness have been noted between older and younger women.

Dose
IBS-C:
290 mcg orally once daily

Chronic constipation:
72 mcg or 145 mcg orally once daily

How Supplied
Linaclotide is available as 75-mcg, 145-mcg, and 290-mcg capsules for oral use.

Prescribing Considerations
Linaclotide has a **black box warning** for avoiding use among individuals under age 18. There is an increased risk of dehydration, possibly fatal, if used by children. Linaclotide should be stored away from children to avoid accidental ingestion.

Linaclotide should be taken on an empty stomach at least 30 minutes prior to the first meal of the day.

Capsules should be swallowed whole and not chewed or crushed.

A missed dose should not be doubled. It should be taken at the next scheduled time.

Abdominal pain and diarrhea should be reported to a healthcare provider.

Cost: $$$$$

Liraglutide (Saxenda, Victoza)

Therapeutic class: Antidiabetic, anti-obesity

Chemical class: Glucagon-like peptide 1 (GLP-1) agonist. Other drugs in this category include dulaglutide and semaglutide.

Indications
Liraglutide (Victoza) is indicated for the improvement of glycemic control and the prevention of major cardiovascular events for adults with type II diabetes.

Liraglutide (Saxenda) is indicated for chronic weight management for adults with a body mass index (BMI) of 30 kg/m^2 or greater or 27 kg/m^2 or greater in the presence of at least one weight-related comorbid condition such as hypertension, type II diabetes mellitus, or dyslipidemia.

Contraindications
Liraglutide is contraindicated for individuals with a personal or family history of medullary thyroid carcinoma or multiple endocrine neoplasia syndrome type 2.

Liraglutide is not indicated for weight loss during pregnancy.

Liraglutide should not be used by individuals with a serious hypersensitivity reaction to the medication or its components.

Mechanism of Action
GLP-1 is a physiological regulator of appetite and calorie intake, and the GLP-1 receptor is present in several areas of the brain involved in appetite regulation. Liraglutide lowers body weight through decreased calorie intake. It does not increase 24-hour energy expenditure.

Metabolism & Excretion
Hepatic and renal

Adverse Reactions
Serious adverse reactions are possible and include acute cholecystitis, acute pancreatitis, acute renal failure, hypoglycemia, increases in heart rate, suicidal ideation, and thyroid C-cell tumors.

Side Effects
Gastrointestinal (GI) side effects are common and include abdominal pain, bloating, constipation, diarrhea, dyspepsia, flatulence, nausea, and vomiting. Dizziness, fatigue, headache, and injection-site discomfort and redness may also occur.

Drug–Drug Interactions
Liraglutide causes delayed gastric emptying and therefore has the potential to affect the absorption of concomitantly administered oral medications.

Specific Considerations for Women
Pregnancy
Liraglutide for weight loss is contraindicated during pregnancy because weight loss is not recommended during pregnancy. There is limited information on the use of liraglutide for glucose control during pregnancy and, based on animal studies, the potential for fetal harm exists. The American College of Obstetricians and Gynecologists (ACOG) and the American Diabetes Association (ADA) continue to recommend human insulin as the standard of care for women diagnosed with gestational diabetes mellitus (GDM) who require medical treatment beyond dietary changes.

Breastfeeding
It is not known if liraglutide is excreted into human milk. Liraglutide is a large peptide molecule, and therefore the amount in breast milk is likely to be very low. Additionally, absorption is unlikely because any ingested drug is probably destroyed in the infant's gastrointestinal tract. Nonpharmacologic methods of weight control should be used by women who are breastfeeding. If glucose control is necessary during lactation, other oral antidiabetic medications or insulin should be considered.

Adolescent women
Safety and effectiveness have not been established for individuals under age 18.

Elderly women
No differences in safety or effectiveness have been noted between older and younger women.

Dose

For weight loss:

3 mg once daily, injected subcutaneously (SQ) into the abdomen, thigh, or upper arm. The dose escalation schedule is as follows:

> Week 1: 0.6 mg
> Week 2: 1.2 mg
> Week 3: 1.8 mg
> Week 4: 2.4 mg
> Week 5 and thereafter: 3 mg

For glucose control:

Initial dose is 0.6 mg once daily, injected SQ into the abdomen, thigh, or upper arm. After one week the dose may be increased to 1.2 mg. The maximum dose for glucose control is 1.8 mg.

How Supplied

Liraglutide is supplied as prefilled, multidose pens for SQ injection.

For weight loss:

Each individual pen delivers doses of 0.6 mg, 1.2 mg, 1.8 mg, 2.4 mg, or 3 mg (6 mg/ml, 3 ml).

For glucose control:

Each individual pen delivers doses of 0.6 mg, 1.2 mg, or 1.8 mg (6 mg/ml, 3 ml).

Prescribing Considerations

Liraglutide has a **black box warning** for risk of thyroid C-cell tumors in mice. Liraglutide should not be prescribed for individuals with a personal or family history of medullary thyroid cancer or for individuals with multiple endocrine neoplasia syndrome type 2.

Liraglutide is marketed under two different brand names for different indications. Saxenda is indicated as an aid for weight loss, and Victoza is indicated for glucose control for individuals with type II diabetes. Doses for each indication are not the same, and providers should exercise caution when prescribing liraglutide.

Weight-loss dose escalations can be delayed a week if GI symptoms occur. However, if the full 3-mg dose cannot be tolerated, the medication should be discontinued as weight-loss efficacy has not been established at lower doses.

Liraglutide pens should be stored in the refrigerator.

Liraglutide should be used as an adjunct to dietary changes and increased exercise for both weight loss and glucose control.

Cost: $$$$$

Lisinopril (Prinivil, Zestril)

Therapeutic class: Antihypertensive

Chemical class: Angiotensin converting enzyme (ACE) inhibitor. Other medications in this class include benazepril, captopril, enalapril, and quinapril.

Indications
Lisinopril is indicated for:

1. Treatment of hypertension (alone or with other antihypertensive agents)
2. Adjunct therapy for the treatment of heart failure
3. Part of a treatment regimen after myocardial infarction

Contraindications
Lisinopril is contraindicated for individuals with a history of angioedema during previous treatment with an ACE inhibitor, those who are hypersensitive to the medication, and for individuals with hereditary or idiopathic angioedema.

Mechanism of Action
Lisinopril inhibits ACE and suppresses the renin-angiotensin-aldosterone system. This results in decreased vasopressor activity and aldosterone secretion.

Metabolism & Excretion
Not metabolized; excreted unchanged in urine

Adverse Reactions
Angioedema can occur at any time during treatment with ACE inhibitors, including lisinopril.

Lisinopril may cause changes in renal function, hyperkalemia, hypotension, and leukopenia.

Side Effects
Cough, dizziness, headache

Drug–Drug Interactions
Concomitant administration with diuretics may increase the potential for hypotension, and use with potassium-sparing diuretics may increase serum potassium.

Concomitant administration of lisinopril with antidiabetic medicines (insulins, oral hypoglycemic agents) may increase the potential for hypoglycemia.

Concomitant use of lisinopril and nonsteroidal anti-inflammatory drugs (NSAIDs) by individuals with renal failure may worsen renal function.

Lisinopril may increase the risk of lithium toxicity.

Specific Considerations for Women
Pregnancy
Lisinopril and other ACE inhibitors are contraindicated during pregnancy. When taken in the second and third trimesters, ACE inhibitors can cause fetal harm or death. If a woman becomes pregnant while taking lisinopril, she should discontinue the medication as soon as pregnancy is discovered.

Breastfeeding
There is no information on lisinopril and breastfeeding. Other ACE inhibitors such as benazepril, captopril, enalapril, and quinapril are excreted in low levels in breast milk and not expected to cause adverse effects for infants who are breastfeeding. These may be alternate medications to consider.

Adolescent women
Lisinopril can be used by adolescent women. The safety and efficacy of lisinopril have been established for individuals beginning at age 6.

Elderly women
There is no evidence to suggest that women over age 65 respond differently than younger women, and no dose adjustments are recommended. In general, doses for individuals who are older should always start at the lowest dosing range and be increased gradually as needed for therapeutic effect.

Dose: Variable, depending on condition being treated
Hypertension:
For uncomplicated hypertension, the initial recommended starting dose is 10 mg orally once per day. The usual dose ranges from 20 mg to 40 mg once daily. If hypertension is not adequately controlled with lisinopril monotherapy, a low-dose diuretic can be added, such as hydrochlorothiazide 12.5 mg.

Heart failure:
For heart failure, lisinopril is often used as adjuvant therapy with digitalis and diuretics. The recommended starting dose is 5 mg orally once per day. The usual dose ranges from 5 mg to 40 mg once per day. Doses should be increased by no more than 10 mg, and at least 2 weeks should elapse between dose changes.

Acute myocardial infarction:
Lisinopril is initiated 24 hours after acute MI for individuals who are hemodynamically stable. Initial starting dose is 5 mg orally, followed by 5 mg in 24 hours, 10 mg after 48 hours, and continuing with 10 mg daily. If systolic blood pressure is low (less than 120 mmHg), then a lower oral dose of 2.5 mg should be given, and the maintenance dose can be lowered to 5 mg once daily.

Dose reductions are indicated for individuals with renal impairment. Complete prescribing information should be reviewed for dosing recommendations.

How Supplied
Lisinopril is supplied in tablets of 2.5-mg, 5-mg, 10-mg, 20-mg, and 40-mg for oral use.

Prescribing Considerations
Lisinopril has a **black box warning** for use during pregnancy. Women of reproductive age who are sexually active and taking lisinopril should be counseled about the importance of using consistent, reliable contraception to avoid an unintended pregnancy. Women who are taking lisinopril and wish to become pregnant should speak with their healthcare provider about transitioning to a medication that is compatible with pregnancy.

A persistent, nonproductive cough is a potential side effect with all ACE inhibitors, including lisinopril. Cough resolves when the medication is discontinued.

Other ACE inhibitors are available that may have a different dosing schedule and cost. Choice of medication should be individualized to the specific needs of each woman.

Cost: $

Lorazepam (Ativan)

Therapeutic class: Anti-anxiety

Chemical class: Benzodiazepine. Other medications in this category include alprazolam, clonazepam, and diazepam.

Indications
Lorazepam is indicated for the management of anxiety disorders or for the short-term relief of anxiety.

Contraindications
Lorazepam is contraindicated for individuals with hypersensitivity to benzodiazepines and for individuals with narrow-angle glaucoma.

Mechanism of Action
Benzodiazepines, including lorazepam, act on the limbic, thalamic, and hypothalamic regions of the central nervous system (CNS) to produce CNS depression, including anticonvulsant activity, hypnosis, sedation, and skeletal muscle relaxation. Benzodiazepines block cortical and limbic arousal that occurs following stimulation of the reticular pathways.

Metabolism & Excretion
Hepatic and renal

Adverse Reactions
Preexisting depression may worsen with use of lorazepam.

Benzodiazepines, including lorazepam, have been associated with physical and psychologic dependence.

Side Effects
Confusion, dizziness, drowsiness, fatigue, paradoxical reactions, sedation, unsteadiness, weakness

Drug–Drug Interactions
Use with opioids increases the risk for fatal respiratory depression. Use with other CNS depressants, such as alcohol, anesthetics, anticonvulsants, antidepressants, antipsychotics, anxiolytics, barbiturates, opioid analgesics, sedative antihistamines, and sedative/hypnotics increases the risk for sedation.

Probenecid and valproate increase the effects of lorazepam.

Specific Considerations for Women
Pregnancy
Emerging research has suggested a possible link between first-trimester use of benzodiazepines and increased risk of spontaneous pregnancy loss. Additionally, benzodiazepine withdrawal symptoms have been observed with infants exposed to benzodiazepines in utero. Nonpharmacologic methods to relieve anxiety are recommended during pregnancy. If women who are taking lorazepam become pregnant, they should taper off the medication.

Breastfeeding
Lorazepam is excreted in low levels in breast milk, and no adverse effects have been noted for infants. Women taking lorazepam may breastfeed.

Adolescent women
Lorazepam may be used by adolescent women. Risks of dependence and adverse neuropsychiatric symptoms, such as paradoxical reactions, should be weighed against the need for the medication.

Elderly women
There is no evidence that older and younger individuals respond differently to lorazepam. However, the risk for sedation and unsteadiness increases with age. Individuals who are older may be at an increased risk for falls. Dose reductions are recommended.

Dose
For the treatment of anxiety, an initial dose of 2 to 3 mg orally per day is given in divided doses two or three times per day. This can be increased as necessary. The usual maximum dose per day is 6 mg. For individuals who are elderly, doses should be reduced to 1 to 2 mg orally per day.

For insomnia related to anxiety, 2 to 4 mg may be given orally at bedtime.

How Supplied
Lorazepam is supplied as 0.5-mg, 1-mg, and 2-mg tablets for oral use.

Prescribing Considerations
Lorazepam has a **black box warning** for the concomitant use of benzo-diazepines with opioids. This combination may result in increased seda-tion, respiratory depression, coma, and death. Women are at increased risk of respiratory depression when taking both benzodiazepines and opioids.

Lorazepam should not be prescribed to manage anxiety associated with everyday life events.

Initial treatment should be limited to 2 to 4 weeks and total treatment should be limited to 4 months. Need for lorazepam beyond this time should be evaluated individually. Risk for physical and psychologic dependence increases with higher doses and longer length of treatment.

Lorazepam is a schedule IV controlled substance. Individuals should be assessed for risk for dependence prior to beginning treatment.

Withdrawal symptoms may occur with abrupt discontinuation. Gradual dose tapering should be used when discontinuing treatment.

Activities that require mental alertness, such as driving, should be avoided until it is known how lorazepam will affect the individual.

Other benzodiazepines are available that may have a different dosing schedule and cost. Choice of medication should be individualized to the specific needs of each woman.

Cost: $

Lorcaserin (Belviq, Belviq XR)

Therapeutic class: Anti-obesity

Chemical class: Serotonin 2C receptor agonist

Indications
Lorcaserin is indicated for chronic weight management for adults with a body mass index (BMI) of 30 kg/m^2 or greater or 27 kg/m^2 or greater in the presence of at least one weight-related comorbid condition such as dyslipidemia, hypertension, or type II diabetes mellitus.

Contraindications
Lorcaserin is not indicated for weight loss during pregnancy.

Lorcaserin should not be used by individuals with a serious hypersensitivity reaction to the medication or its components.

Lorcaserin should not be used in combination with serotonergic and dopaminergic drugs that are potent 5-HT2B receptor agonists and are known to increase the risk for cardiac valvular disease.

Mechanism of Action
The exact mechanism of action is unknown, but lorcaserin is thought to decrease food intake and promote satiety through selective activation of 5-HT2C receptors on anorexigenic neurons in the hypothalamus.

Metabolism & Excretion
Hepatic and renal

Adverse Reactions
Lorcaserin is a serotonergic drug. Potentially fatal neuroleptic malignant syndrome or serotonin syndrome have been reported with serotonergic drugs.

Regurgitant cardiac valvular disease (primarily mitral and/or aortic valves) has been reported by individuals taking serotonergic drugs with 5-HT2B receptor agonist activity.

Other potential adverse reactions include bradycardia, cognitive impairment (attention and memory), confusion, decreases in red and white blood cell counts, elevated prolactin levels, hypoglycemia when used with other hypoglycemic agents, psychiatric symptoms, and pulmonary hypertension.

Side Effects
Constipation, diarrhea, dizziness, dry mouth, fatigue, headache, and nausea may occur.

Drug–Drug Interactions
Due to the potential for serotonin syndrome, lorcaserin should be used cautiously with other serotonergic drugs, including bupropion, dextromethorphan, lithium, monoamine oxidase inhibitors (MAOIs), selective serotonin-norepinephrine reuptake inhibitors (SNRIs), selective serotonin reuptake inhibitors (SSRIs), St. John's wort, tramadol, tricyclic antidepressants (TCAs), triptans, and tryptophan.

Lorcaserin can increase the exposure of drugs that are CYP2D6 substrates.

Specific Considerations for Women
Pregnancy
Lorcaserin is contraindicated during pregnancy because weight loss is not recommended during pregnancy. Maternal weight gain should be based on pre-pregnancy BMI.

Breastfeeding
It is not known if lorcaserin is excreted into human milk. Nonpharmacologic methods of weight management should be used by women who are breastfeeding.

Adolescent women
The safety and efficacy of lorcaserin has not been established for individuals under age 18.

Elderly women
It is unknown if individuals who are older respond differently to lorcaserin compared with younger individuals. Individuals who are elderly and have normal renal function do not require a dose adjustment.

Dose
Lorcaserin 10 mg orally twice daily or lorcaserin extended-release 20 mg orally once daily

How Supplied
Lorcaserin is supplied as 10-mg and 20-mg (extended-release) tablets for oral use.

Prescribing Considerations
Lorcaserin is listed on Schedule IV of the Controlled Substances Act. Euphoria is possible at supratherapeutic doses. Lorcaserin should be prescribed with caution for individuals with a substance abuse history.

Extended-release tablets should not be chewed or crushed.

Response to therapy should be evaluated after 12 weeks. If a 5% loss of body weight has not occurred during this time, it is unlikely that continuing lorcaserin will be beneficial, so the medication should be discontinued.

Symptoms of serotonin syndrome should be reviewed; if they occur, a healthcare provider should be notified immediately.

Lorcaserin should be used as an adjunct to dietary changes and increased exercise for weight loss.

Cost: $$$$$

Medroxyprogesterone acetate (Provera)

Therapeutic class: Endocrine-metabolic agent

Chemical class: Progestin

Indications
Medroxyprogesterone acetate (MPA) is indicated for the treatment of secondary amenorrhea and abnormal uterine bleeding due to hormonal imbalance in the absence of organic pathology, such as fibroids or uterine cancer. MPA is also indicated for use in the prevention of endometrial hyperplasia for women with an intact uterus who are postmenopausal and receiving daily oral conjugated estrogen 0.625-mg tablets.

Contraindications
MPA is contraindicated with:

1. Undiagnosed abnormal vaginal bleeding
2. Known, suspected, or history of breast cancer
3. Known or suspected estrogen or progesterone-dependent neoplasia
4. Active deep vein thrombosis (DVT), pulmonary embolism (PE), or a history of these conditions
5. Active arterial thromboembolic disease, such as stroke or myocardial infarction (MI), or a history of these conditions
6. Known anaphylactic reaction, angioedema, or hypersensitivity to MPA
7. Known liver impairment or disease
8. Known or suspected pregnancy

Mechanism of Action
MPA binds to progesterone receptors and slows the frequency of release of gonadotropin releasing hormone (GnRH) from the hypothalamus and decreases the pre-ovulatory luteinizing hormone (LH) surge.

Metabolism & Excretion
Hepatic and renal

Adverse Reactions

Many of the reported adverse reactions have occurred during daily use of estrogen plus progesterone. It is unclear if the same risks exist for intermittent or daily use of progesterone only.

Potentially serious adverse reactions include abnormal vaginal bleeding; breast, endometrial, and ovarian cancers; cardiovascular disorders; dementia; depression; elevated blood pressure and lipids; hepatic impairment; and visual changes.

Side Effects

Abdominal pain, acne, bloating, breast tenderness, fatigue, hair loss, headache, weight gain

Drug–Drug Interactions

MPA is metabolized via CYP3A4. Specific drug–drug interaction studies evaluating the clinical effects of CYP3A4 inducers or inhibitors on MPA have not been conducted. However, inducers and/or inhibitors of CYP3A4 may affect the metabolism of MPA.

Specific Considerations for Women

M

Pregnancy

MPA is contraindicated during pregnancy. The conditions for which it is used do not occur during pregnancy, and therefore MPA provides no therapeutic benefit to women who are pregnant. Additionally, there may be an increased risk of hypospadias for infants who are male, and clitoral enlargement and labial fusion for infants who are female when exposed to MPA during the first trimester.

Breastfeeding

Oral MPA is excreted in breast milk. Most information on lactation is the result of research on depot medroxyprogesterone acetate (DMPA) contraceptive injection. DMPA has not been found to adversely affect the composition of milk, the growth and development of the infant, or the milk supply.

Adolescent women
Oral MPA has not been well studied among the pediatric population. Irregular menses and secondary amenorrhea are common among adolescents. All options to treat these conditions should be considered.

Elderly women
No differences in safety or effectiveness have been noted between older and younger women. There may be an increased risk of dementia for women over age 65 when MPA is used with estrogen.

Dose
Secondary amenorrhea:
Treatment may be started at any time. Usual dose is 10 mg of MPA orally every day for 10 days, although 5 mg per day can be used. In the presence of adequate estrogen, progestin withdrawal bleeding typically begins within 3 to 7 days after stopping MPA.

Abnormal uterine bleeding:
Treatment is started on the calculated 16th or 21st day of the menstrual cycle. Usual dose is 10 mg orally every day for 5 to 10 days, although 5 mg per day can be used. Optimal response is often seen with 10 mg MPA for 10 days beginning on the 16th day of the cycle. In the presence of adequate estrogen, progestin withdrawal bleeding typically begins within 3 to 7 days after stopping MPA. Women who have a history of recurrent abnormal uterine bleeding may benefit from planned menstrual cycling with MPA.

Reduction of endometrial hyperplasia for women with
an intact uterus using estrogen therapy:
Oral MPA may be given in doses of 5 mg or 10 mg daily for 12 to 14 consecutive days per month, for women who are postmenopausal and receiving daily 0.625-mg conjugated estrogens, either beginning on the first day of the cycle or the 16th day of the cycle.

How Supplied
MPA is supplied as 2.5-mg, 5-mg, and 10-mg tablets for oral use.

Prescribing Considerations

MPA has a **black box warning** for the possibility of breast cancer, cardiovascular events, and dementia when used with estrogen.

Abnormal vaginal bleeding should be reported to a healthcare provider and investigated appropriately.

The lowest dose for the shortest amount of time is prudent.

Cost: $

Mefenamic acid (Ponstel)

Therapeutic class: Analgesic and anti-inflammatory

Chemical class: Anthranilic acid derivative; member of the fenamate group of nonsteroidal anti-inflammatory drugs (NSAIDs). Other NSAIDs include ibuprofen, indomethacin, and naproxen.

Indications

Mefenamic acid is indicated for the treatment of primary dysmenorrhea and for the relief of mild to moderate pain.

Contraindications

Mefenamic acid is contraindicated with active ulceration or chronic inflammation of the gastrointestinal (GI) tract, allergic or anaphylactic reaction to other NSAIDs, aspirin-sensitive asthma, and known hypersensitivity to mefenamic acid.

Mefenamic acid should not be given for the treatment of perioperative pain in the setting of coronary artery bypass graft (CABG) surgery.

Concomitant administration of mefenamic acid and other NSAIDs or salicylates should be avoided due to the increased risk of GI bleeding.

Mechanism of Action

Mefenamic acid is involved in the inhibition of cyclooxygenase and prostaglandin synthesis. This may decrease inflammation and prostaglandin levels in peripheral tissues.

Metabolism & Excretion
Hepatic and renal

Adverse Reactions
Anaphylactic reactions have been reported with NSAIDs.

NSAIDs may increase the risk of serious cardiovascular and thrombotic events, including myocardial infarction (MI) and stroke.

Other adverse reactions can include anemia, edema, elevated liver enzymes, fluid retention, GI bleeding, GI ulcers, heart failure, hepatotoxicity, hyperkalemia, hypertension, and skin reactions.

Side Effects
GI effects are common and include dyspepsia, nausea, pain, and vomiting.

Drug–Drug Interactions
Risk of bleeding may be increased with concomitant use of mefenamic acid and anticoagulants, aspirin, and selective serotonin reuptake inhibitors (SSRIs).

Risk of adverse GI events may be increased with concomitant use of mefenamic acid with aspirin or other NSAIDs.

Mefenamic acid may reduce the effect of angiotensin converting enzyme (ACE) inhibitors, angiotensin receptor blockers (ARBs), beta-blockers, loop and thiazide diuretics.

Mefenamic acid may increase serum concentrations of digoxin and lithium. The risk of methotrexate toxicity and nephrotoxicity with cyclosporine is increased when these medications are used with mefenamic acid.

Specific Considerations for Women
Pregnancy
Mefenamic acid may cause premature closure of the fetal ductus arteriosus. NSAIDs, including mefenamic acid, should not be taken by women who are pregnant starting at 30 weeks of gestation.

Breastfeeding
Only limited information is available about the effects of mefenamic acid on breastfeeding. Other options to consider include acetaminophen, ibuprofen, and naproxen.

Adolescent women

Mefenamic acid may be used to treat primary dysmenorrhea for adolescent women over age 14.

Elderly women

It is unknown if women over age 65 respond differently to mefenamic acid compared with younger women. However, women who are postmenopausal do not have a menstrual cycle and would not need treatment for dysmenorrhea. Individuals who are elderly and use mefenamic acid for general pain conditions are at greater risk of NSAID-related adverse reactions. The lowest dose for the shortest amount of time should be considered.

Dose

The recommended dose for the treatment of primary dysmenorrhea is 500 mg orally as an initial dose, followed by 250 mg orally every 6 hours. Mefenamic acid should be initiated with the onset of menses. Duration of treatment is 2 to 3 days.

The recommended dose for the treatment of acute pain is 500 mg orally as an initial dose, followed by 250 mg orally every 6 hours. Treatment should be limited to no longer than 7 days.

How Supplied

Mefenamic acid is supplied as 250-mg capsules for oral use.

Prescribing Considerations

Mefenamic acid has a **black box warning** for the risk of serious GI events (bleeding, perforation, ulceration) and for an increased risk of cardiovascular and thrombotic events (MI, stroke).

Women taking mefenamic acid for dysmenorrhea should take this medication only when needed to relieve uterine cramping and limit use to 2 to 3 days during the menstrual cycle.

Taking mefenamic acid with food may help decrease the risk of GI upset.

Other NSAIDs are available that may have a different dosing schedule and cost. Choice of medication should be individualized to the specific needs of each woman.

Cost: $$

Metformin hydrochloride, Metformin ER (Fortamet, Glucophage, Glucophage XR, Glumetza, Riomet)

Therapeutic class: Antihyperglycemic

Chemical class: Biguanide

Indications

Metformin is indicated as an adjunct to diet and exercise to improve glycemic control for individuals 10 years of age and older with type II diabetes mellitus. It is often used as an adjunct treatment for polycystic ovary syndrome (PCOS), although it is not approved for the treatment of PCOS or prediabetes.

Contraindications

Metformin is contraindicated with:

1. Severe renal impairment (eGFR below 30 ml/min/1.73 m^2)
2. Acute or chronic metabolic acidosis, including diabetic ketoacidosis, with or without coma
3. Hypersensitivity to metformin

Mechanism of Action

Metformin decreases hepatic glucose production, decreases intestinal absorption of glucose, and improves insulin sensitivity by increasing peripheral glucose uptake and utilization. Metformin also may improve glucose use by adipose tissue and skeletal muscle by increasing glucose transport across cell membranes.

Metabolism & Excretion

Not metabolized; excreted unchanged in the urine

Adverse Reactions

Metformin decreases liver uptake of lactate, which may increase the risk of lactic acidosis (see Prescribing Considerations). It may also decrease vitamin B12 levels.

Side Effects

Gastrointestinal (GI) side effects are common and include abdominal pain, diarrhea, flatulence, nausea, and vomiting.

Drug–Drug Interactions

Use of metformin with insulin and sulfonylurea medications increases the risk of hypoglycemia.

Concomitant use of metformin with carbonic anhydrase inhibitors, including acetazolamide, dichlorphenamide, topiramate, or zonisamide, may increase the risk for lactic acidosis.

Concomitant use of drugs that interfere with the renal elimination of metformin, including cimetidine, dolutegravir, ranolazine, and vandetanib, could increase metformin levels and may increase the risk for lactic acidosis.

Alcohol use with metformin increases the risk of lactic acidosis.

Medications such as calcium channel blockers, corticosteroids, estrogens, isoniazid, nicotinic acid, oral contraceptives, phenothiazines, phenytoin, sympathomimetics, thiazide and other diuretics, and thyroid drugs may increase the risk of hyperglycemia.

Specific Considerations for Women

Pregnancy

Metformin can be used during pregnancy, and it does not appear to increase the risk of birth defects above the national baseline for all pregnancies. The American College of Obstetricians and Gynecologists (ACOG) and the American Diabetes Association (ADA) continue to recommend human insulin as the standard of care for women diagnosed with gestational diabetes mellitus (GDM) who require treatment beyond dietary changes. Per ACOG, metformin may be considered the preferred second-line choice for women who decline insulin therapy, are unable to safely administer insulin, or cannot afford insulin.

Breastfeeding

Metformin is excreted in human breast milk. Package labeling advises women not to breastfeed while taking metformin or to consider risk/benefit and possible infant exposure to the medication. Although hypoglycemia or other side effects are possible for the infant, limited studies have not documented any adverse effects for the infant who is breastfeeding. Infants typically receive less than 0.5% of their mother's weight-adjusted dosage. However, metformin should be used with caution while breastfeeding premature infants.

Adolescent women
Metformin can be used by adolescent women.

Elderly women
No differences in safety or effectiveness have been noted between older and younger women. However, women who are 65 and older are at increased risk of lactic acidosis.

Dose
The starting dose for metformin is 500 mg orally twice a day or 850 mg once a day, with meals. Doses can be increased in increments of 500 mg weekly or 850 mg every 2 weeks, up to a maximum dose of 2,550 mg per day, given in divided doses.

The starting dose for metformin ER is 500 mg orally once daily with dinner. Doses can be increased in increments of 500 mg weekly, up to a maximum of 2,000 mg once daily with dinner.

How Supplied
Metformin is supplied as 500-mg, 850-mg, and 1,000-mg tablets for oral use.

Metformin extended-release (ER) is supplied as 500-mg and 750-mg tablets for oral use.

Prescribing Considerations
Metformin has a **black box warning** for the risk of lactic acidosis that has resulted in bradycardia, death, hypotension, and hypothermia. The risk of lactic acidosis is increased for individuals with renal impairment and/or hepatic impairment, those aged 65 and older, those who have received radiologic studies with contrast, and individuals with excessive alcohol intake. See Contraindications and Interactions. Warning signs

of lactic acidosis (abdominal pain, increased somnolence, malaise, myalgias, respiratory distress) should be discussed with all individuals; if these symptoms occur, metformin should be discontinued and the healthcare provider notified.

Estimated glomerular filtration rate (eGFR) should be assessed prior to treatment and at least annually. See full prescribing information for details on dosing for individuals with renal impairment.

Women who are anovulatory may ovulate after improvement in glucose and insulin resistance with metformin treatment. Contraception should be used if women are not seeking pregnancy.

Hematologic parameters should be assessed annually and vitamin B12 either annually or at least every 2 to 3 years.

Extended-release tablets should not be chewed, crushed, or cut.

Alcohol should be avoided or greatly minimized.

Monitor HgbA1C every three months for response to therapy.

Taking metformin with food may decrease GI side effects.

Cost: $–$$

M

Methadone (Dolophine)

Therapeutic class: Analgesic

Chemical class: Opioid

Indications

Methadone is indicated for:

1. The treatment of moderate to severe pain not responsive to non-narcotic analgesics
2. Detoxification treatment of opioid addiction (heroin or other morphine-like drugs)
3. Maintenance treatment of opioid addiction (heroin or other morphine-like drugs), in conjunction with appropriate social and medical services

Contraindications
Methadone is contraindicated with a known allergy or hypersensitivity to the medication.

Methadone is contraindicated in any situation where opioids are contraindicated (acute bronchial asthma, hypercarbia, or respiratory depression). Methadone should not be used by any individual who has, or is suspected of having, a paralytic ileus.

Mechanism of Action
Methadone is a mu-agonist with multiple actions qualitatively similar to those of morphine that involve the central nervous system (CNS) and organs composed of smooth muscle.

Metabolism & Excretion
Hepatic and renal

Adverse Reactions
Respiratory depression is the main and potentially fatal hazard associated with methadone. The peak respiratory depressant effect of the drug typically occurs later and persists longer than its peak analgesic effects, especially during the initial dosing period. These characteristics can contribute to cases of iatrogenic overdose, particularly during treatment initiation or dose titration.

Methadone inhibits cardiac potassium channels and prolongs the QT interval. QT interval prolongation and serious arrhythmias (torsades de pointes) have been observed during treatment with methadone, especially with higher doses (more than 200 mg per day).

Side Effects
Constipation, dizziness, drowsiness, nausea, sedation, vomiting

Drug–Drug Interactions
Individuals who are tolerant to other opioids may be incompletely tolerant to methadone. Incomplete cross-tolerance is concerning due to the complexity of determining safe dosing during opioid treatment conversion. Deaths have been reported during conversion from chronic, high-dose treatment with other opioid agonists.

Methadone should be administered with extreme caution to individuals with conditions accompanied by decreased respiratory reserve, hypercapnia, or hypoxia, such as asthma, chronic obstructive pulmonary disease (COPD), cor pulmonale, kyphoscoliosis, myxedema, severe obesity, and sleep apnea.

Concomitant administration of methadone with other CNS depressants, such as alcohol, hypnotics, opioids, phenothiazines, sedatives, and tranquilizers increases the risk for respiratory depression.

Concomitant use of methadone and benzodiazepines increases the risk of fatal respiratory depression.

Methadone is metabolized via cytochrome P450 enzymes, principally CYP3A4, CYP2B6, and CYP2C19, and to a lesser extent by CYP2C9 and CYP2D6. Co-administration of methadone with CYP inducers of these enzymes may result in a more rapid metabolism and potential for decreased effects of methadone. Administration with CYP inhibitors may reduce metabolism and potentiate methadone's effects.

Individuals maintained on methadone may experience withdrawal symptoms when given opioid antagonists, mixed agonist/antagonists, and partial agonists.

Pharmacodynamic interactions may occur with concomitant use of methadone and potentially arrhythmogenic agents such as antiarrhythmics, calcium channel blockers, and some neuroleptics and tricyclic antidepressants.

Specific Considerations for Women

Pregnancy

Maternal use of methadone during pregnancy as part of supervised medication-assisted treatment (MAT) for opioid addiction is unlikely to pose a substantial teratogenic risk; however, it is impossible to state that there is no risk. Women who are pregnant and involved in methadone maintenance programs have demonstrated significantly improved prenatal care, leading to a reduced incidence of obstetric and fetal complications and decreased neonatal morbidity and mortality when compared to women using illicit drugs. Methadone clearance can be increased during pregnancy. Women who are pregnant and receiving MAT may need dose adjustments.

There is a high likelihood of neonatal abstinence syndrome (NAS) in the newborn, which may need to be treated pharmacologically.

Breastfeeding
The recommendation for use during breastfeeding varies. Women who received methadone as part of MAT during pregnancy and are stable on this therapy should be encouraged to breastfeed if possible. Methadone may cause respiratory depression and sedation for infants who are breastfeeding and were not exposed to the drug during pregnancy. Therefore, other medications should be considered for pain control postdelivery.

Adolescent women
Safety and efficacy have not been established for individuals under age 18.

Elderly women
No differences in safety or effectiveness have been noted between older and younger women. However, methadone should be used with caution by individuals who are elderly and known to be sensitive to CNS depressants. Individuals who are older often have comorbid conditions and may be taking concomitant medications that could predispose them to developing dysrhythmias.

Dose
Initiation of therapy for individuals who are opioid nontolerant:
The starting dose of methadone is 2.5 mg to 10 mg orally every 8 to 12 hours, slowly titrated to effect.

Conversion to methadone from other chronic opioids:
Can be complex; refer to medication prescribing information for equianalgesic conversion chart.

Detoxification and maintenance treatment of opiate dependence:
The initial methadone dose should be administered, under supervision, when there are no signs of intoxication or sedation and when symptoms of withdrawal are present. A single oral dose of 20 mg to 30 mg of methadone often suppresses withdrawal symptoms. Dose adjustments should

be made over the first week of treatment based on control of withdrawal symptoms at the time of expected peak activity, which occurs 2 to 4 hours after dosing.

Maintenance treatment:
Clinical stability is often achieved at doses between 80 mg to 120 mg per day.

How Supplied
Methadone is supplied as 5-mg and 10-mg tablets for oral use.

Prescribing Considerations
Methadone has a **black box warning** for the risk of death due to cardiac and respiratory depression. Additionally, QT interval prolongation and serious arrhythmias (torsades de pointes) have been associated with the use of methadone.

Methadone is a Schedule II controlled substance with a high potential for abuse and diversion. Abuse of methadone increases the risk of overdose and death.

Methadone for the treatment of opioid addiction in detoxification or maintenance programs can only be dispensed in oral form by opioid treatment programs certified by the Substance Abuse and Mental Health Services Administration and approved by the designated state authority. Methadone for the treatment of opioid addiction cannot be prescribed in an outpatient setting that is not part of an opioid treatment program.

There are many potential drug interactions that can increase the adverse effects of methadone. A complete medication history is essential prior to prescribing additional medications for individuals taking methadone.

Abrupt discontinuation of methadone will result in opioid withdrawal symptoms.

Methadone may impair mental and physical function, and activities that require mental alertness should be avoided until it is known how methadone will affect the individual's functioning.

Cost: $$$–$$$$$

Methylergonovine (Methergine)

Therapeutic class: Oxytocic

Chemical class: Semi-synthetic ergot alkaloid

Indications
Methylergonovine is indicated for the treatment of postpartum hemorrhage related to uterine atony following delivery of the placenta and subinvolution of the uterus. It is also indicated for control of uterine hemorrhage in the second stage of labor following delivery of the anterior shoulder.

Contraindications
Methylergonovine should not be given during pregnancy prior to delivery. It is contraindicated for women with eclampsia, preeclampsia, or significant hypertension or for women with known hypersensitivity to methylergonovine.

Mechanism of Action
Methylergonovine acts directly on the smooth muscle of the uterus and increases the tone, rate, and amplitude of rhythmic contractions. The tetanic uterotonic effect shortens the third stage of labor and reduces blood loss.

Metabolism & Excretion
Hepatic and gastrointestinal (fecal)

Adverse Reactions
Hypertension can occur. There are been rare reports of cardiac disorders, including angina, myocardial infarction, tachycardia, and ventricular fibrillation.

Side Effects
Nausea, painful uterine contractions, vomiting

Drug–Drug Interactions
Beta blockers may enhance the vasoconstrictive effects of methylergonovine.
    CYP3A4 inhibitors: Co-administration of other ergot alkaloid drugs and strong CYP3A4 inhibitors has been linked to vasospasm causing cerebral ischemia. Potent CYP3A4 inhibitors such as azole antifungals, HIV

protease or reverse transcriptase inhibitors, and macrolide antibiotics should be avoided during treatment with methylergonovine.

CYP3A4 inducers: Strong CYP3A4 inducers such as nevirapine and rifampicin may decrease the effectiveness of methylergonovine.

Specific Considerations for Women

Pregnancy

Methylergonovine is a uterotonic and contraindicated during pregnancy. It is indicated for use after delivery.

Breastfeeding

Methylergonovine is excreted in breast milk and may reduce the quantity and quality of milk. Adverse effects for the infant, including irritability and tachycardia, have been reported when women have taken multiple repeated doses. Product labeling advises women to delay breastfeeding for 12 hours after the last administration of methylergonovine. However, single or limited doses of methylergonovine after delivery, prior to the establishment of mature milk, are not expected to transfer appreciable amounts of drug to the infant via colostrum or to increase adverse effects for the infant.

Adolescent women

Methylergonovine can be used by adolescent women to treat postpartum hemorrhage.

Elderly women

Methylergonovine is indicated for the treatment of postpartum hemorrhage and is therefore contraindicated for women who are postmenopausal.

Dose

Oral:

One 0.2-mg tablet, 3 or 4 times daily after delivery for a maximum of 1 week.

Intramuscular (IM):

A 1-ml ampule of 0.2 mg of methylergonovine either after delivery of the anterior shoulder, after delivery of the placenta, or during the immediate postpartum period. Can be repeated as required for uterine atony and hemorrhage, at intervals of 2 to 4 hours.

Intravenous (IV):
Routine administration is not recommended and should only be considered in life-threatening situations due to the possibility of sudden hypertensive and cerebrovascular accidents. IV administration must occur slowly over the course of 60 seconds with continuous blood pressure monitoring.

How Supplied
Methylergonovine is available in 1-ml ampules that contain 0.2 mg methylergonovine maleate for IM or IV injection.

It is also available in 0.2-mg tablets for oral use.

Prescribing Considerations
An expected effect of methylergonovine is strong and potentially painful uterine contractions. Acetaminophen or nonsteroidal anti-inflammatory drugs (NSAIDs) can be taken to alleviate discomfort.

Blood pressure should be monitored during treatment.

Cost: $$–$$$

Metronidazole (Flagyl)

Therapeutic class: Antiprotozoal

Chemical class: Nitroimidazole derivative. Other medications in this category include secnidazole and tinidazole.

Indications
Metronidazole is indicated for the treatment of:

1. Symptomatic and asymptomatic trichomoniasis (*T. vaginalis* infection), including in sexual partners
2. Bacterial vaginosis (BV)
3. Acute intestinal amebiasis (amebic dysentery) and amebic liver abscess
4. Infections caused by susceptible anaerobic bacteria, including gynecologic infections

Contraindications

Metronidazole is contraindicated for individuals with a prior history of hypersensitivity to metronidazole or other nitroimidazole derivatives.

Metronidazole should not be used by individuals who have taken disulfiram within the past 2 weeks due to the possibility of psychotic reactions when the medications are taken together.

Use of oral metronidazole is associated with a disulfiram-like reaction to alcohol, including abdominal cramps, flushing, headaches, nausea, and vomiting. Metronidazole should not be taken with alcohol or products containing propylene glycol during treatment and for at least 24 hours (and up to 72 hours) after treatment is finished.

Mechanism of Action

Metronidazole exerts antibacterial effects in an anaerobic environment against most obligate anaerobes. Metronidazole undergoes intracellular chemical reduction during anaerobic metabolism. After this process, it damages the cell DNA helical structure and breaks its strands, which inhibits bacterial nucleic acid synthesis and causes cell death.

Metabolism & Excretion

Hepatic and renal

M

Adverse Reactions

Cases of encephalopathy and peripheral neuropathy (including optic neuropathy) have been reported with metronidazole. Aseptic meningitis and convulsive seizures have occurred.

Side Effects

Gastrointestinal (GI) upset (abdominal cramping, nausea, vomiting), metallic taste in the mouth, rashes

Drug–Drug Interactions

Alcohol and disulfiram (see Contraindications).

Metronidazole can potentiate the anticoagulant effect of warfarin and other oral coumarin anticoagulants, which can prolong prothrombin time.

Metronidazole may increase the serum concentration of busulfan and lithium.

Drugs that inhibit CYP450 enzymes, such as cimetidine, may prolong the half-life and decrease plasma clearance of metronidazole.

Drugs that induce CYP450 enzymes, such as phenobarbital or phenytoin, may increase the elimination of metronidazole and reduce plasma levels.

Specific Considerations for Women
Pregnancy
Although package labeling states that metronidazole is contraindicated in the first trimester of pregnancy, according to the Centers for Disease Control and Prevention STD Treatment Guidelines, women with a trichomoniasis infection can be treated with 2 grams of metronidazole in a single dose at any stage of pregnancy.

Breastfeeding
Metronidazole is excreted in breast milk. With maternal oral therapy, infants who are breastfeeding receive metronidazole in doses that are lower than those used to treat infections in infants. Some clinicians advise deferring breastfeeding for 12 to 24 hours following maternal treatment with a single 2-gram dose of metronidazole.

Adolescent women
Metronidazole can be used by adolescent women.

Elderly women
No differences in safety or effectiveness have been noted between older and younger women. Individuals who are older may have decreased liver function and require a dose adjustment.

Dose: Variable, depending on condition being treated
Trichomoniasis:
2 grams orally as a single dose (preferred) or 500 mg orally twice daily for 7 days

BV:
500 mg orally twice daily for 7 days

Acute intestinal amebiasis (acute amebic dysentery):
750 mg orally three times per day for 5 to 10 days

Anaerobic bacterial infections:
For serious anaerobic infections, intravenous metronidazole is usually administered initially.

In the case of severe hepatic impairment, the dose of metronidazole should be reduced by 50%.

How Supplied
Metronidazole is supplied as 250-mg or 500-mg tablets for oral use.

Prescribing Considerations
Metronidazole has a **black box warning** because the drug has been shown to be carcinogenic in mice and rats. How this relates to intermittent use in humans is unknown. Package labeling states that unnecessary use of the drug should be avoided.

Completing the full course of metronidazole is necessary.

Partners of women diagnosed with trichomoniasis must also be treated to prevent reinfection.

Inform women about the interaction of this drug with alcohol.

Taking metronidazole with food may decrease GI side effects.

Women who are HIV-positive and have been diagnosed with trichomoniasis should be treated with metronidazole 500 mg orally twice daily for 7 days (rather than with a 2-gram single dose of metronidazole). Retesting is recommended in 3 months.

Other nitroimidazole medications, such as secnidazole and tinidazole, are available and have a different dosing schedule and cost. Choice of medication should be individualized to the specific needs of each woman.

Cost: $–$$

Metronidazole vaginal gel, 0.75% (Metrogel)

Therapeutic class: Antibiotic and antiprotozoal

Chemical class: Nitroimidazole derivative

Indications
Metronidazole vaginal gel is indicated for the treatment of bacterial vaginosis (BV).

Contraindications
Metronidazole is contraindicated for individuals with a prior history of hypersensitivity to metronidazole, other nitroimidazole derivatives, or parabens.

Disulfiram-like reactions to alcohol have been reported with oral metronidazole; thus, the possibility of such a reaction occurring while using metronidazole vaginal gel therapy cannot be excluded.

Mechanism of Action
The action of metronidazole on anaerobes is not completely known. The 5-nitro group of metronidazole is reduced by metabolically active anaerobes, and the reduced form of the drug interacts with bacterial DNA.

Metabolism & Excretion
Hepatic and renal

Adverse Reactions
Psychotic reactions have occurred among individuals who took oral metronidazole and disulfiram concurrently. Metronidazole vaginal gel should not be used by women who have taken disulfiram within the past 2 weeks.

Cases of encephalopathy and peripheral neuropathy (including optic neuropathy) have been reported with oral metronidazole. If these symptoms appear, metronidazole vaginal gel should be discontinued.

Side Effects
Approximately 10% of women treated with metronidazole vaginal gel developed symptomatic vaginal candidiasis during or immediately after therapy.

Drug–Drug Interactions

Possible disulfiram-like reaction to alcohol (see Contraindications).

Oral metronidazole has been reported to potentiate the anticoagulant effect of warfarin and other oral coumarin anticoagulants and increase the serum concentration of busulfan and lithium. Significantly lower systemic concentrations of metronidazole occur with the vaginal gel, but the possibility of drug interactions cannot be excluded.

Specific Considerations for Women

Pregnancy

Oral metronidazole therapy has not been shown to be superior to topical (vaginal) therapy for treating symptomatic BV during pregnancy. Women who are pregnant and have BV symptoms can use either oral or vaginal metronidazole.

Breastfeeding

Metronidazole is excreted in breast milk. With maternal oral therapy, infants who are breastfeeding receive metronidazole in doses that are lower than those used to treat infections in infants. Some clinicians advise deferring breastfeeding for 12 to 24 hours following maternal treatment with a single 2-gram dose of oral metronidazole. It is expected that systemic absorption of the vaginal gel produces a lower concentration in breast milk, so this form is considered compatible with breastfeeding.

Adolescent women

Metronidazole vaginal gel can be used by adolescent women.

Elderly women

There are no reported differences in response to metronidazole vaginal gel between older and younger women.

Dose

The treatment of BV is metronidazole gel 0.75%, one full applicator (5 grams) intravaginally, once a day for 5 days.

How Supplied

Metronidazole vaginal gel 0.75% is supplied in a 70-gram tube and packaged with 5 vaginal applicators.

Prescribing Considerations
Completing the full 5-day course of metronidazole vaginal gel is necessary, even if symptoms improve or resolve.

Inform women about the possibility of interaction with alcohol.

Women who are HIV-positive and have been diagnosed with BV can receive the same treatment regimen as women who are HIV-negative.

Women should be instructed to abstain from vaginal intercourse during treatment.

Metronidazole vaginal gel can be used during menses, but tampons will absorb the medication and should not be used during treatment.

Metronidazole vaginal gel is supplied with 5 vaginal applicators. For once-daily dosing, one applicator should be used per dose and then discarded, and a new applicator used for the next day's dose. If an applicator must be reused, it should be washed and dried prior to the next use.

Cost: $$

Miconazole vaginal (Monistat and many generics)

Therapeutic class: Antifungal

Chemical class: Imidazole

Indications
Miconazole vaginal is indicated for the treatment of vulvovaginal candidiasis.

Contraindications
Miconazole is contraindicated with hypersensitivity to other azoles.

Mechanism of Action
Miconazole interferes with ergosterol biosynthesis. This alters fungal cell membrane permeability and causes destruction of the cell.

Metabolism & Excretion
Hepatic and renal

Adverse Reactions
No clinically significant adverse reactions have been reported.

Side Effects
The most commonly reported side effects are local burning, irritation, and itching.

Drug–Drug Interactions
There are no known clinically significant drug–drug interactions.

Specific Considerations for Women
Pregnancy
Pregnancy predisposes women to the development of vaginal candidiasis due to changes in the vaginal microbial environment. Miconazole treatment of vaginal candidiasis during pregnancy has not been associated with fetal harm. During pregnancy, azole antifungals such as miconazole should be used in a 7-day formulation.

Breastfeeding
Miconazole has poor oral bioavailability, and it is unlikely to adversely affect infants who are breastfeeding. Topical application to the nipples has been used for the treatment of oral thrush.

Adolescent women
Miconazole can be used by adolescent women.

Elderly women
No differences in safety or effectiveness have been noted between older and younger women.

Dose
Many different over-the-counter (OTC) formulations exist:

Miconazole 2% cream, 5 grams intravaginally daily for 7 days

Miconazole 4% cream, 5 grams intravaginally daily for 3 days

Miconazole 100-mg vaginal suppository, one suppository daily for 7 days

Miconazole 200-mg vaginal suppository, one suppository daily for 3 days

Miconazole 1,200-mg vaginal suppository, one suppository for 1 day

How Supplied
See Dose.

Prescribing Considerations
Miconazole products are available over-the-counter (OTC), and there are many formulations, including 1-, 3-, and 7-day treatment options with either cream or suppositories.

Women can choose the treatment length and type that best fits their needs and lifestyle.

More severe infections, especially for individuals who are immunocompromised, may require longer treatment.

If women don't respond after self-treatment with OTC miconazole, they should be evaluated clinically.

Cost: $

Mifepristone (Mifeprex)

Therapeutic class: Abortifacient

Chemical class: Synthetic steroid, progestin antagonist

Indications
Mifepristone is indicated for the medical termination of intrauterine pregnancy through 70 days gestation when used in combination with misoprostol. Pregnancy is dated from the first day of the last menstrual period (LMP); if LMP is unknown or uncertain, pregnancy dating is per ultrasonography.

Contraindications
Mifepristone (and subsequent misoprostol) is contraindicated with allergy to mifepristone or other prostaglandins, current anticoagulant therapy,

hemorrhagic disorders that could contribute to heavy bleeding, inherited porphyrias, known or suspected ectopic pregnancy, risk of acute renal insufficiency (concurrent long-term corticosteroid therapy or chronic adrenal failure), and undiagnosed adnexal mass.

Mechanism of Action

Mifepristone is a progestin antagonist that inhibits the activity of progesterone. When combined with misoprostol, the effects on the uterus and cervix result in the termination of pregnancy.

Metabolism & Excretion

Hepatic and gastrointestinal (fecal)

Adverse Reactions

Major and potentially fatal adverse events include infection, sepsis, and prolonged, excessive vaginal bleeding (defined as soaking through two thick, full-size sanitary pads per hour for two consecutive hours). Mifepristone has a **black box warning** for these major adverse reactions.

Side Effects

Abdominal pain and cramping (expected), bleeding heavier than a normal menstrual period (expected), diarrhea, dizziness, fever/chills, nausea, vomiting

Drug–Drug Interactions

CYP3A4 inducers: CYP450 3A4 is primarily responsible for the metabolism of mifepristone. CYP3A4 inducers such as dexamethasone, rifampin, St. John's wort, and certain anticonvulsants (such as carbamazepine, phenobarbital, and phenytoin) may increase mifepristone metabolism and potentially lower mifepristone concentrations.

CYP 3A4 inhibitors: Based on the metabolism of mifepristone, CYP3A4 inhibitors such as erythromycin, grapefruit juice, itraconazole, and ketoconazole may inhibit the metabolism of mifepristone, resulting in increased serum concentrations. Mifepristone should be used with caution by women currently or recently treated with a CYP3A4 inhibitor.

Specific Considerations for Women
Pregnancy
Mifepristone, in combination with misoprostol, is indicated for the termination of pregnancy and should not be taken by women who wish to continue a
pregnancy. In cases of failed termination, there could be disruption of early
embryonic or fetal development. Birth defects have been reported after a
failed termination of pregnancy using mifepristone and misoprostol.

Breastfeeding
Mifepristone is excreted in breast milk in low levels. Women may continue
to breastfeed after a single dose of mifepristone.

Adolescent women
Mifepristone is considered safe for adolescent women in the termination of
pregnancy.

Elderly women
Mifepristone, in combination with misoprostol, is indicated for the termination of pregnancy, and thus is not appropriate for women who are
postmenopausal.

Dose
For medical abortion, 200 mg of mifepristone are given orally as a single
dose followed by 800 mcg of misoprostol buccally 24 to 48 hours after
mifepristone.

How Supplied
Mifepristone is supplied on a blister card as a single 200-mg tablet for
oral use.

Prescribing Considerations
Mifepristone has a **black box warning** for possibility of severe or fatal infections and bleeding following mifepristone use during medical abortions.
    Mifepristone can only be prescribed by clinicians who have completed
the Mifeprex Risk Evaluation and Management Strategy (REMS) program.
Healthcare providers must be certified with the program and complete a

Prescriber Agreement Form. Women must also sign a Patient Agreement Form. Mifepristone can be dispensed for women only in certain healthcare settings, clinics, offices, and hospitals by or under the supervision of a certified prescriber. Information on the REMS program is available at 1-877-4 Early Option (1-877-432-7596) or at https://www.earlyoptionpill.com /for-health-professionals/prescribing-mifeprex/

Women who are rhesus (RH) negative should receive Rho(D) immune globulin after medical abortion, to prevent RH isoimmunization.

Women should follow up with their healthcare provider within 7 to 14 days after taking mifepristone and misoprostol to confirm completion of pregnancy termination.

Cost: $$$

Mirabegron (Myrbetriq)

Therapeutic class: Urinary tract antispasmodic

Chemical class: Beta-3 adrenergic agonist

M

Indications
Mirabegron is indicated for the treatment of symptoms of overactive bladder (OAB), including urinary frequency, urinary urge incontinence, and urinary urgency. It can be used as monotherapy or in combination with the muscarinic antagonist solifenacin succinate.

Contraindications
Mirabegron is contraindicated for individuals with hypersensitivity to the drug or components.

Mirabegron should not be prescribed for individuals with severe uncontrolled hypertension (systolic blood pressure greater than or equal to 180 mm Hg and/or diastolic blood pressure greater than or equal to 110 mm Hg) or for individuals with severe hepatic impairment or end-stage renal disease.

Mechanism of Action
Mirabegron increases bladder capacity by relaxing detrusor smooth muscle during the storage phase of the bladder fill-void cycle, which increases bladder capacity.

Metabolism & Excretion
Primarily renal

Adverse Reactions
Potentially serious adverse reactions include angioedema, hypertension, and urinary retention in the presence of bladder outlet obstruction.

Side Effects
Constipation, dizziness, dry mouth, headache, nausea, rash, urinary tract infections, tachycardia

Drug–Drug Interactions
Mirabegron is a moderate CYP2D6 inhibitor. Mirabegron may increase levels of drugs such as desipramine, digoxin, metoprolol, and warfarin.

Specific Considerations for Women
Pregnancy
There are no data on the effects of mirabegron on the developing fetus. Urinary frequency is common during pregnancy, and medications for OAB, including mirabegron, are generally not prescribed.

Breastfeeding
Mirabegron is present in the milk of animals. However, there is no information on the presence of mirabegron in human milk or information on how mirabegron might affect milk quality or quantity.

Adolescent women
There are no safety or efficacy data for women under age 18.

Elderly women
No differences in safety or effectiveness have been noted between older and younger women. No dose adjustments are necessary for women over age 65.

Dose

Monotherapy:

The recommended starting dose of mirabegron is 25 mg orally once daily with or without food. Improvement in symptoms is seen within 8 weeks. The dose may be increased to 50 mg once daily to control symptoms of OAB if the starting dose is ineffective.

Combination therapy:

The recommended starting dose of mirabegron is 25 mg orally once daily with solifenacin succinate 5 mg orally once daily. The mirabegron dose may be increased to 50 mg once daily after 4 to 8 weeks.

How Supplied

Mirabegron is available as 25-mg and 50-mg extended-release tablets for oral use.

Prescribing Considerations

For individuals with moderate hepatic impairment or severe renal impairment, the daily dose should not exceed 25 mg.

Because hypertension is possible, blood pressure should be monitored during treatment. However, the recommended frequency of this assessment hasn't been determined.

Tablets should not be chewed or crushed.

Cost: $$$$$

Misoprostol (Cytotec)

Therapeutic class: Antiulcerative

Chemical class: Synthetic prostaglandin E1 analogue

Indications

Misoprostol is approved for oral administration to prevent gastric ulcers for individuals who take anti-inflammatory drugs on a long-term basis. It is also approved for use in first-trimester medical abortion in conjunction with mifepristone.

It is used off label in other regimens for cervical priming before uterine procedures, such as intrauterine device (IUD) insertion and hysteroscopy, labor induction, prevention and treatment of postpartum hemorrhage, and treatment of early pregnancy loss.

This book focuses on misoprostol in combination with mifepristone for medical abortion.

Contraindications
Misoprostol is contraindicated with hypersensitivity to misoprostol, other prostaglandins, or their analogues. It should not be taken by women who are pregnant and wish to continue the pregnancy.

Mechanism of Action
For a first-trimester medical abortion, misoprostol stimulates uterine contractions and softens the cervix to assist in the expulsion of uterine contents.

Metabolism & Excretion
Hepatic and renal

Adverse Reactions
Adverse reactions are rare when used as part of an approved protocol for medical abortion. Pregnancy loss and uterine rupture have occurred during off-label use and during treatment for gastric ulcers.

Side Effects
The most common side effects associated with misoprostol for medical abortion are abdominal pain, diarrhea, and nausea. Uterine cramping and vaginal bleeding are expected as part of the medical abortion.

Drug–Drug Interactions
There are no documented, major drug–drug interactions when misoprostol is used as a single 800-mcg dose for medical abortion.

Specific Considerations for Women
Pregnancy
Congenital anomalies, including those associated with fetal death, have been reported after unsuccessful use of misoprostol as an abortifacient. However, the teratogenic mechanism of misoprostol is unclear.

Breastfeeding
Misoprostol is excreted in breast milk in extremely low levels. There are no documented reports of adverse effects of misoprostol for infants who are breastfeeding. A single dose of 800 mcg associated with medical abortion is unlikely to affect lactation or cause adverse effects.

Adolescent women
Misoprostol is appropriate for medical termination of pregnancy for women of all reproductive ages.

Elderly women
Women who are postmenopausal are not at risk for pregnancy, and therefore misoprostol is not indicated for pregnancy termination in this group.

Dose
Medical abortion:
800 mcg of misoprostol 24 to 48 hours after mifepristone. Two 200-mcg tablets of misoprostol are placed in each cheek pouch (400 mcg each side, total of 800 mcg) and allowed to dissolve over 30 minutes. Any remaining medication is swallowed.

How Supplied
Misoprostol is available as 100-mcg or 200-mcg tablets.

Prescribing Considerations
Misoprostol has a **black box warning** related to use by women of childbearing age in the treatment of gastric ulcers. If misoprostol is not taken as part of a regimen for medical abortion, it can result in congenital anomalies, pregnancy loss, preterm delivery, and uterine rupture. The medication may

M

also cause uterine rupture when used off label for cervical ripening and induction of labor.

Nonsteroidal anti-inflammatory drugs (NSAIDs) are not contraindicated for women who undergo a medical abortion and are appropriate first-line agents for pain management. NSAIDs inhibit the synthesis of new prostaglandins but do not block the action of prostaglandin receptors. NSAIDs do not inhibit the action of a prostaglandin used for medical abortion.

Women should be advised that they will experience bleeding that is heavier than a regular menstrual period and should expect uterine cramping that may be severe enough to require medication for the discomfort. NSAIDs or acetaminophen are appropriate.

Instruct the woman that excessive bleeding, defined as soaking through two maxipads per hour for 2 consecutive hours, should be reported to the healthcare provider.

Most women will expel the pregnancy within 24 hours after taking misoprostol. They should plan on being in a location in which they can be comfortable and manage the vaginal bleeding.

Women should follow up with their healthcare provider within 7 to 14 days after taking mifepristone and misoprostol to confirm completion of pregnancy termination.

Women who are rhesus (RH) negative should receive Rho(D) immune globulin to prevent RH isoimmunization.

Cost: $–$$

Naloxone hydrochloride nasal spray (Narcan)

Therapeutic class: Narcotic antagonist

Chemical class: Opioid antagonist

Indications
Naloxone nasal spray is indicated for the emergency treatment of a known or suspected opioid overdose manifested by central nervous system (CNS) and respiratory depression.

Contraindications
Naloxone is contraindicated with a known allergy or hypersensitivity.

Mechanism of Action
Naloxone is an opioid antagonist that competes for opioid receptor sites.

Metabolism & Excretion
Hepatic and renal

Adverse Reactions
There is a high likelihood that naloxone will precipitate opioid withdrawal for individuals who are opioid dependent. Symptoms may include abdominal cramps, body aches, diarrhea, fever, irritability, nausea, runny nose, shivering, sneezing, sweating, tachycardia, vomiting, and weakness.

After initial response, respiratory depression may reoccur. Repeat doses and additional respiratory support may be required.

Side Effects
Congestion, edema, headache, hypertension, inflammation and dryness of the nasal passages, musculoskeletal pain

Drug–Drug Interactions
There are no known drug–drug interactions with naloxone. The medication may have limited effectiveness against partial agonists or mixed agonists/antagonists.

Specific Considerations for Women
Pregnancy
Limited data are available on the use of naloxone for women who are pregnant. Animal studies do not suggest embryotoxic or teratogenic effects. It is possible that naloxone could precipitate withdrawal in the fetus, especially if maternal use of opioids has been prolonged and at high doses. Fetal monitoring should occur after naloxone administration for women who are pregnant.

Breastfeeding
Naloxone is not orally bioavailable and is not expected to affect breastfeeding. However, if naloxone was given to treat an opioid overdose, it is prudent to avoid breastfeeding after a large dose of opioids.

Adolescent women
Naloxone can be given to adolescent women experiencing opioid overdose.

Elderly women
No differences in safety or effectiveness have been noted between older and younger women after the administration of naloxone.

Dose
Each single spray delivers 4 mg of naloxone hydrochloride. The entire spray should be administered intranasally in one nostril. Repeat doses may be required.

How Supplied
Naloxone is supplied in a blister package containing two 4-mg single-use doses of naloxone hydrochloride in a 0.1-ml intranasal spray.

Prescribing Considerations
Naloxone will be administered by someone other than the individual with opioid addiction. Those who could administer naloxone should understand that administration should occur as quickly as possible. Prolonged respiratory or CNS depression increases the risk for death.

Emergency medical assistance should be summoned as soon as the overdose is recognized.

Multiple doses may be required and can be administered in alternating nostrils every 2 to 3 minutes.

Cost: $$–$$$

Naltrexone-bupropion (Contrave)

Therapeutic class: Anti-obesity

Chemical class: Opioid antagonist + aminoketone

Indications
Naltrexone-bupropion is indicated as an adjunct to a reduced-calorie diet and increased physical activity for chronic weight management for adults with an initial body mass index (BMI) of: 30 kg/m^2 or greater (obese) *or* 27 kg/m^2 or greater (overweight) in the presence of at least one weight-related comorbid condition such as dyslipidemia, hypertension, or type II diabetes mellitus.

Contraindications
Naltrexone-bupropion is contraindicated for individuals with:

1. Uncontrolled hypertension
2. Seizure disorder or a history of seizures
3. Use of other bupropion-containing products
4. Bulimia or anorexia nervosa, which increase the risk for seizure
5. Chronic opioid or opiate agonist (methadone) or partial agonist (buprenorphine) use, or acute opiate withdrawal
6. Abrupt discontinuation of alcohol, antiepileptic drugs, barbiturates, or benzodiazepines
7. Concomitant administration of monoamine oxidase inhibitors (MAOIs) or use within 14 days
8. Known allergy to bupropion, naltrexone, or any other component of the medication
9. Pregnancy

Mechanism of Action
Naltrexone is an opioid antagonist, and bupropion is a weak inhibitor of the neuronal reuptake of dopamine and norepinephrine. The exact mechanism of action for weight loss is not fully understood, but data suggest that naltrexone and bupropion have effects on two separate areas of the brain involved in the regulation of food intake. The hypothalamus regulates appetitie, and the mesolimbic dopamine circuit regulates the reward system.

Metabolism & Excretion
Hepatic and renal

Adverse Reactions
Potentially serious adverse reactions include aggression; agitation; allergic and anaphylactic reactions; anxiety; central nervous system (CNS) and neuropsychiatric symptoms of psychosis, delusions, hallucinations, hepatotoxicity, homicidal ideation, hostility, hypertension, narrow-angle glaucoma, panic, paranoia, seizures, suicidal thoughts and behaviors; and tachycardia.

Side Effects
Constipation, diarrhea, dizziness, dry mouth, headache, hot flushes, insomnia, nausea

Drug–Drug Interactions
Co-administration of naltrexone-bupropion with high-fat meals results in a significant increase in systemic exposure of naltrexone-bupropion.

Individuals taking naltrexone-bupropion may not fully benefit from treatment with opioid-containing medicines, including antidiarrheal medications, cough remedies, and opioid analgesics. Naltrexone-bupropion should be temporarily discontinued for individuals requiring intermittent opioid treatment.

Bupropion is primarily metabolized by CYP2B6. Bupropion may interact with drugs that are inhibitors or inducers of CYP2B6. Clopidogrel and ticlopidine may increase bupropion levels. Carbamazepine, efavirenz, lopinavir, phenobarbital, phenytoin, and ritonavir may decrease bupropion levels.

Other drug interactions exist. Full prescribing information should be consulted.

Specific Considerations for Women
Pregnancy
Naltrexone-bupropion is contraindicated during pregnancy because weight loss is not recommended and could cause fetal harm. There are no consistent data indicating that either medication causes definite fetal harm during the first trimester. If a woman becomes pregnant while taking naltrexone-bupropion, the medication should be discontinued.

Breastfeeding
There is no information on combination use of naltrexone-bupropion during breastfeeding. Each individual medication is excreted in breast milk in small amounts. Medications to promote weight loss are generally not recommended during lactation. Nonpharmacologic interventions, such as dietary and lifestyle modifications, are the first-line modalities for weight control while breastfeeding.

Adolescent women
There are no safety data on the use of naltrexone-bupropion by women under age 18.

Elderly women
No differences in safety or effectiveness have been noted between older and younger women. However, individuals who are older may be more sensitive to the adverse CNS effects of naltrexone-bupropion. This medication is primarily excreted by the kidneys, and the risk of adverse reactions may be greater for individuals with impaired renal function, which is more common among the elderly.

Dose
The dose of naltrexone-bupropion is increased over the course of 4 weeks:
    Week 1: 1 tablet orally in the morning
    Week 2: 1 tablet orally in the morning and 1 in the evening
    Week 3: 2 tablets orally in the morning and 1 in the evening
    Week 4: 2 tablets orally in the morning and 2 tablets in the evening

Dose adjustments:
Hepatic impairment: maximum dose is 1 tablet in the morning
    Moderate to severe renal impairment: maximum dose is 1 tablet in the morning and 1 in the evening

How Supplied
Naltrexone-bupropion is supplied as 8 mg of naltrexone hydrochloride and 90 mg of bupropion hydrochloride in a fixed-dose extended-release tablet for oral use.

Prescribing Considerations

Naltrexone-bupropion has a **black box warning** for the possibility of suicidal thoughts and behaviors and neuropsychiatric reactions. Individuals and their family members should report any symptoms of aggressiveness, agitation, akathisia, anxiety, hostility, hypomania, impulsivity, insomnia, irritability, mania, or panic attacks.

Tablets should not be chewed, crushed, or cut. Naltrexone-bupropion should not be taken with a high-fat meal.

Response to treatment should be evaluated after 12 weeks at the maintenance dose (2 tablets twice daily). If an individual has not lost at least 5% of baseline body weight, it is unlikely that clinically meaningful weight loss will be reached or sustained, and treatment should be discontinued.

Blood pressure should be monitored during treatment.

At least 14 days should elapse between discontinuation of an MAOI for treatment of depression and beginning treatment with naltrexone-bupropion. Conversely, at least 14 days should be allowed after stopping naltrexone-bupropion before starting an MAOI antidepressant.

An opioid-free interval of a minimum of 7 to 10 days is recommended for individuals previously dependent on short-acting opioids, and those transitioning from buprenorphine or methadone may need as long as 2 weeks.

Prior to initiating treatment with bupropion, individuals should be screened for bipolar disorder to reduce the risk of inducing a mixed/manic episode.

Cost: $$$$$

Nitrofurantoin (Furadantin, Macrobid, Macrodantin)

Therapeutic class: Urinary tract anti-infective

Chemical class: Nitrofurantoin

Indications
Nitrofurantoin is indicated for the treatment of acute, uncomplicated urinary tract infections (UTIs) caused by susceptible strains of *Escherichia coli* or *Staphylococcus saprophyticus*.

Contraindications
Nitrofurantoin is contraindicated with anuria, clinically significant elevated serum creatinine, creatinine clearance under 60 ml per minute, or oliguria.

Although nitrofurantoin is used broadly during pregnancy, it is contraindicated for women who are pregnant at term (38 weeks and beyond), during labor and delivery, or when the onset of labor is imminent. This is due to the possibility of hemolytic anemia for the infant from immature erythrocyte enzyme systems.

Nitrofurantoin should not be used by individuals with glucose-6-phosphate dehydrogenase (G6PD) deficiency due to the increased risk of hemolysis.

Mechanism of Action
Nitrofurantoin inhibits bacterial cell wall synthesis and is bactericidal in urine at therapeutic doses.

Metabolism & Excretion
Hepatic and renal

Adverse Reactions
Acute and chronic pulmonary reactions have occurred as well as hemolytic anemia and neuropathy.

Clostridium difficile-associated diarrhea (CDAD) has been reported with use of nearly all antibacterial agents, including nitrofurantoin.

Side Effects
Diarrhea, flatulence, headache, nausea

Drug–Drug Interactions
Antacids containing magnesium trisilicate reduce the absorption of nitrofurantoin.

Uricosuric drugs, such as probenecid and sulfinpyrazone, can inhibit renal secretion of nitrofurantoin and result in toxic levels.

Specific Considerations for Women

Pregnancy

Nitrofurantoin may be used during pregnancy and is a preferred antibiotic for uncomplicated UTIs during pregnancy. It should not be used at term or during labor.

Breastfeeding

Nitrofurantoin is excreted in breast milk in small amounts. It should not be used by women who are breastfeeding if their infant is less than 8 days old or if their infant has G6PD deficiency due to the risk for hemolysis. Women who are breastfeeding older infants (more than 8 days old) may take nitrofurantoin.

Adolescent women

Adolescent women may take nitrofurantoin.

Elderly women

No differences in safety or effectiveness have been noted between older and younger women. Individuals who are older are more likely to have impaired renal function, and nitrofurantoin is contraindicated with a creatinine clearance less than 60 ml per minute or a significantly elevated serum creatinine.

Dose

Macrodantin: 50 mg to 100 mg orally four times daily for 7 days

   Macrobid: 100 mg orally twice daily for 7 days

How Supplied

Nitrofurantoin is supplied as 25-mg, 50-mg, and 100-mg capsules for oral use.

Prescribing Considerations

Taking nitrofurantoin with food will decrease GI side effects.

   All medication should be finished even if symptoms resolve.

   To reduce the risk of resistance, nitrofurantoin should be given only if a UTI is confirmed by culture or strongly suspected.

Cost: $$

Omeprazole (Prilosec)

Therapeutic class: Gastric acid suppressor

Chemical class: Proton pump inhibitor (PPI). Other medications in this category include esomeprazole, lansoprazole, pantoprazole, and rabeprazole.

Indications
Omeprazole is indicated for the treatment of:
1. Duodenal and gastric ulcer for adults
2. Gastroesophageal reflux disease (GERD) for adults and children
3. Maintenance of healing of erosive esophagitis

Contraindications
Omeprazole is contraindicated with a known hypersensitivity to the medication or to benzimidazole.

Concomitant use of atazanavir and PPIs is not recommended. Co-administration of atazanavir with omeprazole is expected to substantially decrease atazanavir plasma concentrations and reduce the therapeutic effect.

Mechanism of Action
Omeprazole suppresses gastric acid secretion by specific inhibition of the $H+ /K+$ ATPase enzyme system at the secretory surface of the gastric parietal cell. This blocks the first step in acid secretion.

Metabolism & Excretion
Hepatic and renal

Adverse Reactions
Atrophic gastritis on biopsy has been seen with long-term use of omeprazole.

Use with amoxicillin and/or clarithromycin as part of dual or triple therapy must consider the adverse reactions associated with those antibiotics.

Side Effects
Abdominal pain, diarrhea, flatulence, headache, nausea, vomiting

Drug–Drug Interactions

Omeprazole can prolong the elimination of diazepam, phenytoin, and warfarin.

Drugs metabolized by cytochrome P450 may be affected when taken concurrently with omeprazole.

Concomitant administration of omeprazole and tacrolimus may increase the serum levels of tacrolimus.

Specific Considerations for Women

Pregnancy

Evidence from epidemiologic data and retrospective research does not indicate that the use of PPIs during pregnancy increases the risk for major congenital birth defects, spontaneous abortions, or preterm delivery. Dietary changes are considered a first-line approach for treating GERD caused by an enlarged uterus.

Breastfeeding

Limited data indicate that maternal omeprazole doses of 20 mg daily produce low levels in milk. This amount is not expected to cause any adverse effects for infants who are breastfeeding.

Adolescent women

Omeprazole is approved for pediatric use and can be used by adolescent women.

Elderly women

No differences in safety or effectiveness have been noted between older and younger women. There are no recommended dose adjustments for individuals over age 65.

Dose: Variable, depending on condition being treated

Short-term treatment of active duodenal ulcer:

20 mg orally once daily for 4 to 8 weeks

H. pylori *eradication for duodenal ulcer risk reduction:*

Triple therapy (omeprazole/clarithromycin/amoxicillin): Omeprazole 20 mg/clarithromycin 500 mg/amoxicillin 1,000 mg each given orally twice daily for 10 days

Dual therapy: Omeprazole 40 mg orally once daily plus clarithromycin 500 mg three times daily for 14 days

Gastric ulcer:
40 mg orally once daily for 4 to 8 weeks

GERD:
20 mg orally once daily for 4 weeks, extended to 8 weeks in the presence of erosive esophagitis

Healing of erosive esophagitis:
20 mg orally once daily

Pathological hypersecretory conditions:
20 mg orally once daily; may be increased, but doses above 80 mg per day should be divided

How Supplied
Omeprazole is available as a capsule or caplet in doses of 10 mg, 20 mg, and 40 mg. The 40-mg strength requires a prescription.

Prescribing Considerations
In the treatment of GERD, dietary and lifestyle changes should be implemented in addition to omeprazole therapy.

A growing body of research evidence suggests that long-term use of PPIs is associated with a decrease in bone mineral density (BMD). However, there are no evidence-based guidelines beyond suggested treatment duration to guide use. Women taking a PPI, including omeprazole, should be aware of the possible association between PPIs and BMD decrease, and individual risk for fracture should be considered during treatment.

A growing body of research evidence also suggests that use of PPIs increases the risk of *Clostridium difficile* infection, especially among hospitalized individuals. How this risk might affect individuals who are community-dwelling and using PPIs intermittently is not known.

Other PPIs are available that have different doses and cost. Choice of medication should be individualized to the specific needs of each woman.

Cost: $–$$

Ondansetron (Zofran)

Therapeutic class: Antiemetic

Chemical class: Serotonin 5-HT3 receptor antagonist

Indications
Ondansetron is indicated for the treatment of nausea and vomiting associated with:

1. Postoperative nausea and/or vomiting
2. Cancer chemotherapy that is highly emetogenic or initial/repeat courses that are moderately emetogenic
3. Radiotherapy for individuals receiving either total body irradiation, single high-dose fraction to the abdomen, or daily fractions to the abdomen

Ondansetron has been used off label to treat nausea and vomiting of pregnancy (NVP), and nausea and vomiting associated with acute gastroenteritis and other illnesses.

Contraindications
Ondansetron is contraindicated with known hypersensitivity to the medication. It should not be given concurrently with apomorphine due to the risk of hypotension and loss of consciousness.

Mechanism of Action
Ondansetron is a selective 5-HT3 receptor antagonist. Serotonin receptors of the 5-HT3 type are present both peripherally on vagal nerve terminals and centrally in the chemoreceptor trigger zone of the area postrema. Ondansetron's antiemetic action may be mediated centrally, peripherally, or in both sites.

Metabolism & Excretion
Hepatic

Adverse Reactions
Anaphylaxis, bronchospasm, and hypersensitivity reactions have been reported by individuals with a hypersensitivity to other selective 5-HT3 receptor antagonists.

Electrocardiogram (ECG) changes, including QT interval prolongation, have occurred.

The development of serotonin syndrome has been reported with use of 5-HT3 receptor antagonists.

It is possible that postoperative use of ondansetron may mask an ileus or gastric distension.

Side Effects

Constipation, drowsiness, fatigue, headache

Drug–Drug Interactions

Serotonin syndrome is possible if ondansetron is used concomitantly with other serotonergic drugs.

Ondansetron is metabolized by hepatic cytochrome P450 drug-metabolizing enzymes (CYP3A4, CYP2D6, CYP1A2). Inducers or inhibitors of these enzymes may change the clearance and half-life of ondansetron.

Specific Considerations for Women

Pregnancy

NVP should first be managed with nonpharmacologic measures. If modifications to diet and lifestyle are ineffective, the first-line pharmacologic treatment is doxylamine succinate/pyridoxine hydrochloride. Ondansetron has been used off label as a treatment for NVP and hyperemesis unresponsive to other measures. Associations of cleft palate and renal agenesis among fetuses exposed to ondansetron during the first trimester have been suggested. These possible associations must be weighed against the known adverse effects of untreated and unrefractory vomiting during pregnancy.

Breastfeeding

No adverse effects have been reported for infants who are breastfeeding, and ondansetron has been used for infants. Ondansetron is often used for postoperative nausea for women who have a surgical birth. Limited duration of use during lactation is not expected to cause any adverse effects for infants.

Adolescent women

Adolescent women may use ondansetron. It is approved for use by children.

Elderly women
No differences in safety and effectiveness have been observed between older and younger individuals taking ondansetron.

Dose
Doses of 4 mg or 8 mg orally two to three times per day are typical if using the medication off label for various short-term illnesses associated with nausea and vomiting.

To decrease postoperative nausea and vomiting, 16 mg are administered 1 hour before induction of anesthesia.

Clearance is reduced for individuals with severe hepatic impairment. A total daily dose of 8 mg should not be exceeded if severe hepatic impairment is present.

How Supplied
Ondansetron is available as 4-mg and 8-mg oral tablets and oral disintegrating tablets.

Prescribing Considerations
The extent and rate of absorption are greater for women than men. Slower clearance by women, a smaller volume of distribution, and higher absolute bioavailability may result in higher plasma concentrations for women. These factors should be considered when determining doses.

Ondansetron may cause dizziness or drowsiness. Activities that require mental alertness, such as driving, should be avoided until women know how ondansetron may affect them.

Cost: $–$$

Oseltamivir phosphate (Tamiflu)

Therapeutic class: Antiviral

Chemical class: Neuraminidase inhibitor. Other drugs in this category include peramivir and zanamivir.

Indications
Oseltamivir is indicated for treatment of acute, uncomplicated illness due to influenza A and B infection for infants 2 weeks of age and older, children, and adults who have been symptomatic for no more than 48 hours. It is also indicated for the prophylaxis of influenza A and B infection for individuals age 1 year and older.

Contraindications
Oseltamivir is contraindicated for individuals with known serious hypersensitivity to oseltamivir or any component of the product.

Mechanism of Action
Oseltamivir is an inhibitor of influenza virus neuraminidase affecting the release of viral particles.

Metabolism & Excretion
Hepatic and renal

Adverse Reactions
Anaphylaxis and serious skin reactions, including Stevens-Johnson syndrome (SJS) and erythema multiforme, have been reported.

Delirium and other neuropsychiatric events have been reported, although the extent to which these symptoms can be attributed to oseltamivir or the influenza infection cannot be determined.

Side Effects
Diarrhea, headache, nausea, vomiting

Drug–Drug Interactions
Oseltamivir can be administered without regard to the timing of the inactive influenza vaccine. The live influenza nasal vaccine should not be administered concurrently with oseltamivir (see Prescribing Considerations).

Specific Considerations for Women
Pregnancy
There are no well-controlled studies of oseltamivir use by women who are pregnant, but available data do not suggest an increased risk of birth defects.

Women who are pregnant are at higher risk of severe complications from influenza, which may lead to adverse maternal and fetal outcomes including birth defects, low birth weight and infants who are small for gestational age, maternal death, preterm delivery, and stillbirth.

Breastfeeding
Oseltamivir and its active metabolite appear to be poorly excreted into breast milk. The low levels in breast milk are not expected to cause any adverse effects for infants who are breastfeeding, especially if the infant is older than 2 months. Infants can receive oseltamivir directly in doses much larger than those expected to appear in breast milk.

Adolescent women
Adolescent women may use oseltamivir. It is approved for use by infants and children.

Elderly women
No differences in safety and effectiveness have been observed between older and younger individuals taking oseltamivir.

Dose
Acute influenza:
The recommended dose of oseltamivir for treatment of influenza A and B for adults and adolescents 13 years of age and older is 75 mg orally twice daily (one 75-mg capsule or 12.5 ml of oral suspension twice daily) for 5 days.

Influenza prophylaxis:
The recommended dose of oseltamivir for prophylaxis of influenza A and B for adults and adolescents 13 years of age and older is 75 mg orally once daily (one 75-mg capsule or 12.5 ml of oral suspension once daily) for at least 10 days following close contact with an individual infected with influenza and up to 6 weeks during a community outbreak. For individuals who are immunocompromised, oseltamivir may be continued for up to 12 weeks. The duration of protection lasts for as long as oseltamivir is continued.

Doses for infants and children under age 13, and for individuals with renal impairment, are detailed in the full prescribing information.

How Supplied
Oseltamivir is supplied as 30-mg, 45-mg, and 75-mg capsules for oral use.

Oseltamivir is also supplied as a powder blend in a glass bottle. After constitution with 55 ml of water, each bottle delivers a usable volume of 60 ml of oral suspension equivalent to 360 mg oseltamivir base (6 mg/ml).

Prescribing Considerations
Oseltamivir is not a substitute for the yearly influenza vaccination.

The clinical benefit of oseltamivir is variable and dependent on many factors, such as age, presence of comorbid conditions, timing of treatment initiation, type of influenza virus, and viral virulence.

Oseltamivir may reduce the effectiveness of intranasal live attenuated influenza vaccine (LAIV). Oseltamivir should not be given 2 weeks prior to or for 48 hours after administration of the LAIV.

Cost: $$$$

Ospemifene (Osphena)

Therapeutic class: Endocrine-metabolic agent

Chemical class: Estrogen agonist/antagonist; selective estrogen receptor modulator (SERM)

Indications
Ospemifene is indicated for the treatment of moderate to severe dyspareunia due to vulvovaginal atrophy associated with menopause.

Contraindications
Ospemifene is contraindicated for women who are pregnant. It is also contraindicated for women with:

1.   Undiagnosed vaginal bleeding

2. Known or suspected estrogen-related neoplasia
3. Current or history of cerebral vascular accident (CVA), deep vein thrombosis (DVT), myocardial infarction (MI), and/or pulmonary embolism (PE)

Mechanism of Action
Ospemifene is an estrogen agonist/antagonist with tissue-selective effects. Ospemifene binds to estrogen receptors, which activates estrogenic pathways in some tissues (agonism) and blocks estrogenic pathways in others (antagonism).

Metabolism & Excretion
Hepatic and gastrointestinal (fecal)

Adverse Reactions
Ospemifene may increase the risk of CVA, DVT, endometrial carcinoma, endometrial hyperplasia, MI, and PE.

Side Effects
Increased perspiration, increased vaginal discharge, vasomotor symptoms (hot flushes/flashes)

Drug–Drug Interactions
Ospemifene is primarily metabolized by CYP3A4 and CYP2C9.

Fluconazole (strong CYP2C9 inhibitor) and ketoconazole (strong CYP3A4 inhibitor) both increase the systemic exposure of ospemifene.

Rifampin (strong CYP3A4 and moderate CYP2C9 inducer) decreases the systemic exposure of ospemifene.

Specific Considerations for Women
Pregnancy
Ospemifene causes fetal harm and should not be taken by women who are pregnant or who may become pregnant. Embryo-fetal lethality has occurred in animal models.

Breastfeeding
Ospemifene should not be used for dyspareunia related to breastfeeding. It is not known if ospemifene is excreted in breast milk or if there are any adverse effects on the infant who is breastfeeding.

Adolescent women
Adolescent women are not menopausal, and ospemifene is not indicated for this population.

Elderly women
No differences in safety or effectiveness have been noted between older and younger women. There are no age-related dose adjustments for postmenopausal women who are older.

Dose
One 60-mg tablet orally daily with food.

How Supplied
Ospemifene is supplied as a 60-mg tablet for oral use.

Prescribing Considerations
Ospemifene has a **black box warning** for an increased risk of endometrial cancer, endometrial hyperplasia, and thromboembolic events.

Women who are postmenopausal and are taking ospemifene need to report any episodes of vaginal bleeding, and diagnostic measures such as endometrial biopsy should be considered to rule out malignancy.

Adding a progestin to ospemifene for women who are postmenopausal with an intact uterus can be considered, especially if treatment is prolonged.

Ospemifene may induce or potentiate vasomotor symptoms for some women.

It is unknown how ospemifene affects women with current or previous breast cancer and is not recommended for this population.

Cost: $$$$$

Oxytocin (Pitocin)

Therapeutic class: Oxytocic

Chemical class: Exogenous hormone

Indications
Oxytocin is indicated for the initiation or improvement of uterine contractions to achieve vaginal delivery. In this setting, it is indicated for:

1. Induction of labor for women with a medical indication for the initiation of labor
2. Stimulation or reinforcement of labor
3. As adjunctive therapy in the management of incomplete or inevitable abortion, especially during the second trimester

Oxytocin is also indicated after delivery to produce uterine contractions during the third stage of labor and to control postpartum bleeding or hemorrhage.

Contraindications
According to product labeling, antepartum use of oxytocin is contraindicated in any of the following circumstances:

1. Cephalopelvic disproportion, unfavorable fetal positions or presentations that are undeliverable without conversion prior to delivery
2. Obstetrical emergencies where the benefit-to-risk ratio for either the fetus or the mother favors surgical birth
3. Fetal distress where vaginal birth is not imminent
4. Where adequate uterine activity fails to achieve satisfactory progress
5. When the uterus is already hyperactive or hypertonic
6. Where vaginal birth is contraindicated (active genital herpes, cord prolapse, total placenta previa, vasa previa)
7. Women with hypersensitivity to the drug

Mechanism of Action
Oxytocin has specific receptors in the myometrium, and administration results in uterine contractility.

Metabolism & Excretion
Hepatic and renal

Adverse Reactions
Uterine hyperstimulation can produce hypertonic and/or tetanic contractions that may result in cervical and vaginal lacerations, fetal hypoxia, postpartum hemorrhage, precipitous labor, uterine rupture, uteroplacental hypoperfusion, and variable deceleration of the fetal heart rate.

Oxytocin has an antidiuretic effect and could result in water intoxication.

Side Effects
Oxytocin can result in strong and painful contractions.

Drug–Drug Interactions
Severe hypertension has been reported when oxytocin was given 3 to 4 hours following prophylactic administration of a vasoconstrictor in conjunction with caudal block anesthesia.

Oxytocin used with cyclopropane anesthesia may produce maternal hypotension and bradycardia with abnormal atrioventricular rhythms.

Specific Considerations for Women
Pregnancy
Other than augmentation of labor, oxytocin is only indicated for use in pregnancy during a spontaneous or induced abortion. However, it is not expected to present a risk of fetal abnormalities.

Breastfeeding
Oxytocin is a natural hormone. Women who receive oxytocin for the augmentation of labor or as a treatment for uterine atony may breastfeed.

Adolescent women
Adolescent women can receive oxytocin for the augmentation of labor or as a treatment for uterine atony.

Elderly women
There is no therapeutic benefit from administering oxytocin to women who are postmenopausal.

Dose

Initiation or augmentation of labor:

Ten units (1 ml) of oxytocin is added to 1,000 ml of intravenous (IV) solution such as lactated Ringers or 0.9% sodium chloride. The initial dose should be 0.5 to 1 mU/min (equal to 3 to 6 ml of the dilute oxytocin solution per hour). At 30- to 60-minute intervals, the dose should be gradually increased in increments of 1 to 2 mU/min until the desired contraction pattern has been established. Once the desired frequency of contractions has been reached and labor has progressed to 5 to 6 cm dilation, the dose may be reduced by similar increments.

Control of postpartum bleeding:

Oxytocin in doses of 10 to 40 units may be added to 1,000 ml of IV solution. Infusion rate is adjusted to control uterine atony.

or

Oxytocin can be administered by intramuscular (IM) injection in a dose of 10 units of oxytocin (1 ml) after delivery of the placenta.

How Supplied

Oxytocin is supplied in single-use vials of 10 units (1 ml) or in multidose vials of 10 ml, containing 10 units of oxytocin per ml.

Prescribing Considerations

Oxytocin has a **black box warning** stating that it should not be used for elective induction of labor without medical necessity.

An infusion pump is necessary to ensure an accurate rate of infusion when used during labor.

Electronic fetal monitoring should be used at least intermittently to assess fetal heart rate response to contractions. Oxytocin should be discontinued in the presence of fetal distress.

Oxytocin IV infusion should not be administered outside a healthcare setting.

Cost: Limited to no availability in commercial pharmacies

Paroxetine (Brisdelle, Paxil)

Therapeutic class: Antidepressant

Chemical class: Selective serotonin reuptake inhibitor (SSRI)

Indications
Paroxetine (Brisdelle) is indicated for the treatment of moderate to severe vasomotor symptoms (VMS) of menopause.

Paroxetine (Paxil) is indicated for the treatment of generalized anxiety disorder, major depressive disorder (MDD), obsessive compulsive disorder (OCD), panic disorder, post-traumatic stress disorder (PTSD), and social anxiety disorder.

Contraindications
Paroxetine shouldn't be taken with (1) a monoamine oxidase inhibitor (MAOI), due to the increased risk of serotonin syndrome; or (2) thioridazine and pimozide because paroxetine can increase levels of both medications and prolong the QT interval.

Mechanism of Action
The mechanism of action in the reduction of VMS of menopause is unclear. Decreasing estrogen levels associated with menopause may affect the hypothalamus and change both serotonin and norepinephrine levels. This may alter the thermoregulatory set point in the hypothalamus and trigger temperature instability. Paroxetine may reduce vasomotor symptoms through activation of serotonin receptors in the hypothalamus.

The mechanism of action for the treatment of psychiatric conditions is linked to potentiation of serotonergic activity in the central nervous system resulting from inhibition of neuronal reuptake of serotonin (5-hydroxytryptamine, 5-HT). Paroxetine blocks the uptake of serotonin and is a potent and selective inhibitor of serotonin reuptake.

Metabolism & Excretion
Hepatic and renal

Adverse Reactions
In addition to contraindications and adverse events associated with medication interactions, potential serious adverse reactions include akathisia, impaired motor skills, and an increased risk of suicidal thoughts or actions.

Side Effects
Decreased libido, fatigue, headache, insomnia, lethargy, nausea, vomiting

Drug–Drug Interactions
Concomitant use of MAOIs and SSRIs can result in serotonin syndrome. Use of paroxetine and serotonergic drugs such as amphetamines, buspirone, fentanyl, lithium, St. John's wort, tramadol, tricyclic antidepressants (TCAs), triptans, or tryptophan may increase the risk of serotonin syndrome.

Paroxetine is a strong CYP2D6 inhibitor. Paroxetine may increase levels of certain medications such as atomoxetine, pimozide, risperidone, theophylline, thioridazine, tricyclic antidepressants, and warfarin.

Paroxetine may decrease levels of tamoxifen.

Certain medications, including cimetidine, fosamprenavir/ritonavir, phenobarbital, and phenytoin, may decrease levels of paroxetine.

Concomitant use of aspirin, nonsteroidal anti-inflammatory drugs (NSAIDs), warfarin, and other anticoagulants may increase bleeding risk.

Specific Considerations for Women
Pregnancy
Paroxetine (Brisdelle) is contraindicated for women who are pregnant because VMS of menopause do not occur during pregnancy.

Paroxetine (Paxil) may cause fetal harm, including cardiac anomalies, especially when taken during the first trimester. Paroxetine should be avoided during pregnancy and another SSRI, such as sertraline, considered for the treatment of psychiatric conditions.

Breastfeeding
Paroxetine is excreted in breast milk. The amounts ingested by the infant are small, especially in the lower dose used to treat VMS of menopause. If a woman is breastfeeding and experiencing vasomotor symptoms associated with a transition to menopause, she can take paroxetine without interruption

in lactation. When women are taking paroxetine in doses needed to treat psychiatric conditions, the infant who is breastfeeding may have a higher exposure to the drug. Sertraline may be considered as an alternate medication.

Adolescent women
Adolescent women are not menopausal and therefore paroxetine (Brisdelle) is contraindicated for VMS for this population. Adolescent women may take paroxetine (Paxil) for psychiatric conditions if the clinical need outweighs the risks associated with the medication for this age group.

Elderly women
No differences in safety or effectiveness have been noted between older and younger women. No age-related dose adjustment of paroxetine is needed for women who are postmenopausal and taking paroxetine (Brisdelle) for VMS of menopause. Individuals who are older and taking paroxetine (Paxil) for psychiatric conditions may have decreased clearance of the drug, so a lower starting dose (10 mg) is recommended.

Dose
The recommended dose of Brisdelle for VMS of menopause is 7.5 mg orally each day, taken at bedtime.

The recommended dose of Paxil for psychiatric conditions varies depending on the specific condition being treated:

General anxiety disorder:
20 mg orally once daily; may be increased in 10-mg increments up to 50 mg daily

MDD:
20 mg once daily; may be increased in 10-mg amounts up to 50 mg daily

OCD:
40 mg orally once daily, initiated at a dose of 20 mg and increased in 10-mg increments up to 60 mg daily

Panic disorder:
40 mg orally once daily, initiated at a dose of 20 mg and increased in 10-mg increments up to 60 mg daily

PTSD:
20 mg orally once daily; may be increased in 10-mg increments up to 50 mg daily

Social anxiety disorder:
20 mg orally once daily; may be increased in 10-mg increments up to 60 mg daily

How Supplied
Paroxetine (Brisdelle) is supplied as a 7.5-mg capsule for oral use.

Paroxetine (Paxil) is supplied as 10-mg, 20-mg, 30-mg, and 40-mg tablets for oral use.

Prescribing Considerations
Paroxetine has a **black box warning** for an increased risk of suicidal thoughts or behaviors, especially when used by adolescents and young adults. Women and their family members should monitor for agitation, behavior and mood changes, irritability, and suicidality while taking paroxetine.

Paroxetine is available in different strengths and brand names. Prescribers need to be cautious when choosing the correct dose and indication. Brisdelle is marketed for the treatment of VMS of menopause. Paxil is marketed for the treatment of multiple psychiatric conditions.

Brisdelle contains a subtherapeutic dose for treatment of depression, generalized anxiety disorder, or other mental health conditions. Women should not rely on this dose of paroxetine to treat or manage any psychiatric conditions.

Paroxetine for VMS of menopause should not be prescribed for women who are taking another SSRI.

Prior to initiating treatment with an antidepressant, individuals should be screened for bipolar disorder to reduce the risk of inducing a mixed/manic episode.

Paroxetine should not be taken concurrently with an MAOI. A 14-day time period should elapse after stopping an MAOI before beginning paroxetine, and an MAOI shouldn't be started until 14 days after stopping paroxetine.

SSRIs may cause withdrawal symptoms of agitation, headache, and sleep disturbances if stopped abruptly. Although the risk is reduced with a lower dose of paroxetine to treat VMS of menopause, tapering off the medication will reduce the risk of SSRI withdrawal symptoms and worsening of VMS.

Cost: $$–$$$$

Penicillin G benzathine injection (Bicillin LA)

Therapeutic class: Antibiotic

Chemical class: Penicillin

Indications
Intramuscular penicillin G benzathine is indicated for the treatment of:
1. Syphilis
2. Mild-to-moderate upper respiratory tract infections (URIs) due to susceptible streptococci
3. Prophylaxis for rheumatic fever and cholera

Contraindications
Penicillin G is contraindicated for individuals with a previous allergic reaction or hypersensitivity to any penicillin. Penicillin should be used with caution by individuals with a known cephalosporin allergy.

P

Mechanism of Action
Penicillin G exerts a bactericidal action against penicillin-susceptible microorganisms. It renders the bacteria cell wall osmotically unstable.

Metabolism & Excretion
Hepatic and renal

Adverse Reactions
Allergic reactions, including anaphylaxis, are possible.

Clostridium difficile-associated diarrhea (CDAD) has been reported with use of nearly all antibacterial agents, including penicillin.

Side Effects

Antibiotics, including penicillin G, may promote overgrowth of nonsusceptible organisms such as fungi and result in oral thrush or vulvovaginal candidiasis. Other side effects include diarrhea and nausea.

Drug–Drug Interactions

Tetracycline may antagonize the bactericidal effect of penicillin.

Probenecid increases and prolongs serum penicillin levels.

Specific Considerations for Women

Pregnancy

Penicillin G is acceptable for use during pregnancy. Maternal syphilis should be treated to prevent transmission to the fetus. Women who are pregnant, have syphilis, and are allergic to penicillin should undergo desensitization and be treated with penicillin G injection in a supervised setting.

Breastfeeding

Penicillin G is excreted in breast milk in low amounts and not expected to cause adverse effects for the infant. It is compatible with breastfeeding.

Adolescent women

Adolescent women may take penicillin G.

Elderly women

No differences in safety or effectiveness have been reported between older and younger women. Penicillin G is excreted primarily by the kidneys, and individuals who are older are more likely to have impaired renal function.

Dose: Variable, depending on condition being treated

Group A streptococcal URI (streptococcal pharyngitis):
A single injection of 1,200,000 units

Primary, secondary, latent syphilis:
2,400,000 units (2 injections of 1,200,000 units)

Late syphilis (tertiary and neurosyphilis):
2,400,000 units (2 injections of 1,200,000 units) every 7 days for 3 weeks

Prophylaxis for rheumatic fever or cholera:
A single injection of 1,200,000 units once monthly or 600,000 units every 2 weeks

How Supplied
Penicillin G benzathine injectable suspension is supplied in packages of disposable syringes in the following doses:

    1-ml size, containing 600,000 units per syringe
    2-ml size, containing 1,200,000 units per syringe
    4-ml size, containing 2,400,000 units per syringe

Prescribing Considerations
Penicillin G benzathine has a **black box warning** to caution against intravenous (IV) use. Inadvertent IV administration of penicillin G has resulted in cardiac arrest and death.

Penicillin G should be administered by deep IM injection into the dorsogluteal or ventrogluteal muscle.

The Jarisch-Herxheimer reaction occurs for at least half of individuals with early syphilis. The reaction occurs within the first 24 hours after the penicillin injection and manifests as influenza-like symptoms of fever, headache, malaise, and sweating. The reaction is not harmful, and treatment is supportive. Individuals should be warned about the possibility of a Jarisch-Herxheimer reaction and how to manage the symptoms. If a Jarisch-Herxheimer reaction occurs during pregnancy, it may result in fetal distress. Women who are pregnant and treated with penicillin G may require fetal monitoring.

Cost: $$$

Pentosan polysulfate (Elmiron)

Therapeutic class: Urinary analgesic
Chemical class: Carbohydrate derivative

Indications
Pentosan is indicated for the relief of bladder pain and discomfort associated with interstitial cystitis.

Contraindications
Pentosan is contraindicated for individuals with known allergy or hypersensitivity to the product or its compounds.

Mechanism of Action
The exact mechanism of action of pentosan in the treatment of interstitial cystitis is not known. Pentosan is a low-molecular-weight heparin-like compound. It has anticoagulant and fibrinolytic effects and adheres to the bladder wall mucosal membrane. The drug may act as a buffer to control cell permeability and prevent irritating solutes in the urine from reaching the cells.

Metabolism & Excretion
Hepatic and gastrointestinal (fecal)/renal

Adverse Reactions
There are no serious adverse reactions associated with the use of pentosan.

Side Effects
The most commonly observed side effects include abdominal pain, bruising, diarrhea, dyspepsia, hair loss, headache, nausea, rash, and slightly elevated liver enzymes. Pentosan is a weak anticoagulant and could possibly increase bleeding.

Drug–Drug Interactions
Use with other medications that have an anticoagulant effect could increase the risk of bleeding.

Specific Considerations for Women
Pregnancy
There are no adequate, well-controlled studies that included women who are pregnant. Until more data are available, pentosan should not be used during pregnancy.

Breastfeeding
There is no information on pentosan use by women who are breastfeeding.
It is not known if pentosan is excreted in breast milk.

Adolescent women
Safety has been established for adolescent women beginning at age 16.

Elderly women
No differences in safety or effectiveness have been noted between older and
younger women.

Dose
The recommended dose is 100 mg orally three times per day.

How Supplied
Pentosan is supplied as a 100-mg hard gelatin capsule for oral use.

Prescribing Considerations
Pentosan should be taken with water 1 hour prior to or 2 hours after a meal.

   Women should be evaluated after 3 months of treatment. If sufficient
improvement has not occurred, treatment can be extended for an additional
3 months (6 months total). If pain and discomfort have not improved after
6 months, pentosan should be discontinued because it is unlikely that improvement will occur after this point.

   Because pentosan is a weak anticoagulant, concomitant use with aspirin,
other nonsteroidal anti-inflammatory drugs (NSAIDs), or oral anticoagulants may increase bleeding risk.

P

Cost: $$$$$

Permethrin cream, 5% (Elimite)

Therapeutic class: Topical scabicide

Chemical class: Pyrethroid insecticide

Indications
Permethrin cream 5% is indicated for the treatment of scabies.

Contraindications
Permethrin is contraindicated for individuals with a known allergy or hyper-sensitivity to the product.

Mechanism of Action
Permethrin acts on the nerve cell membrane of the insect to disrupt the sodium channel current and cell membrane polarization. Paralysis of the insect occurs.

Metabolism & Excretion
Hepatic and renal

Adverse Reactions
No serious adverse reactions have been associated with the use of topical permethrin.

Side Effects
A scabies infection is often accompanied by edema, erythema, and pruritus. Treatment with permethrin cream can temporarily exacerbate these conditions. The cream may cause burning or stinging.

Drug–Drug Interactions
There are no known drug–drug interactions associated with permethrin products.

Specific Considerations for Women
Pregnancy
There is no evidence of harm to the fetus from topically applied permethrin. If a scabies infection requires treatment during pregnancy, permethrin cream is acceptable.

Breastfeeding
Permethrin cream is acceptable for use by women who are breastfeeding. Less than 2% is absorbed after topical application. Additionally, the medication is rapidly metabolized to inactive metabolites and is safe for direct

use on infant skin. Direct application to the nipple and areola should be avoided.

Adolescent women
Permethrin cream is approved for pediatric use beginning at age 2 months.

Elderly women
No differences in safety or effectiveness have been noted between older and younger women.

Dose
Permethrin cream 5% should be massaged into the skin from the head to the soles of the feet. Scabies rarely infests the scalp of adults, although the forehead, hairline, neck, and temple may be infested among infants and individuals who are elderly, and treatment can be extended to these areas. The cream should be removed by washing (shower or bath) after 8 to 14 hours.

How Supplied
Permethrin cream 5% is available in a 60-gram tube.

Prescribing Considerations
There should be enough cream in one tube for 2 applications for an average adult, although one application is usually curative.

A temporary increase in pruritus is common after application of permethrin and is not typically a sign of treatment failure. Presence of live mites after 14 days requires retreatment.

Permethrin cream and lotion 1% are also available over-the-counter for the treatment of lice. This strength is unlikely to be effective in treating scabies.

Cost: $$

Phenazopyridine (Pyridium, multiple over-the-counter formulations)

Therapeutic class: Urinary analgesic

Chemical class: Diaminopyridine and azo compound

Indications
Phenazopyridine is indicated for the symptomatic relief of burning, frequency, pain, urgency, and other discomforts resulting from irritation of the mucosa of the lower urinary tract caused by infection, surgery, trauma, or urinary tract procedures.

Contraindications
Phenazopyridine should not be used by individuals who have glucose-6-phosphate dehydrogenase (G6PD) deficiency.

Phenazopyridine is contraindicated for individuals with hepatic or renal insufficiency.

Mechanism of Action
Phenazopyridine is excreted in the urine, where it exerts a topical analgesic effect on the mucosa of the lower urinary tract.

Metabolism & Excretion
Hepatic and renal

Adverse Reactions
Hemolytic anemia, methemoglobinemia, and sulfhemoglobinemia are possible, especially in the presence of G6PD.

Side Effects
Phenazopyridine will discolor urine. Diarrhea, headache, nausea, rash, and vomiting are possible.

Drug–Drug Interactions
When given concurrently with ciprofloxacin, phenazopyridine may increase the bioavailability of ciprofloxacin.

Due to dye properties, phenazopyridine may interfere with urinalysis results based on color reactions.

Specific Considerations for Women
Pregnancy
There are no adequate and well-controlled studies involving women who are pregnant. Phenazopyridine should be used by women who are pregnant only if the benefit clearly outweighs potential unknown risks.

Breastfeeding
The safety of phenazopyridine during breastfeeding has not been established. Because it can cause hemolytic anemia, methemoglobinemia, and sulfhemoglobinemia, it should be avoided while breastfeeding.

Adolescent women
Adolescent women may take phenazopyridine at the recommended adult dose.

Elderly women
No differences in safety or effectiveness have been noted between older and younger women. Phenazopyridine may be taken by women over age 65. Consider renal function of individuals who are elderly when choosing the dose.

Dose
The recommended dose is 200 mg orally three times daily with meals. Treatment should be limited to 2 days.

How Supplied
Phenazopyridine is available by prescription in doses of 100-mg and 200-mg tablets for oral use. Over-the-counter formulations contain less than 100 mg of phenazopyridine.

Prescribing Considerations
Phenazopyridine provides symptomatic relief but does not cure urinary infections. It is not a substitute for antibiotics.

Phenazopyridine will discolor body fluids, feces, and urine an orange or red color and may cause staining of skin or clothing.

Taking the medication with food or meals will decrease possible gastrointestinal upset.

Cost: $

Phentermine-topiramate (Qsymia)

Therapeutic class: Anti-obesity

Chemical class: Sympathomimetic amine anorectic + antiepileptic

Indications

Phentermine-topiramate is indicated as an adjunct to a reduced-calorie diet and increased physical activity for chronic weight management for adults with a body mass index (BMI) of:

30 kg/m^2 or greater

or

27 kg/m^2 or greater in the presence of at least one weight-related co-morbid condition such as dyslipidemia, hypertension, or type II diabetes mellitus.

Contraindications

Phentermine-topiramate is contraindicated with:

1. Pregnancy
2. Glaucoma
3. Hyperthyroidism
4. During or within 14 days of taking monoamine oxidase inhibitors (MAOIs)

Mechanism of Action

The effect of phentermine on weight and weight management is likely mediated by release of catecholamines in the hypothalamus, resulting in reduced appetite and decreased food consumption. The effect of topiramate on chronic weight management may be due to its effects on both appetite suppression and satiety enhancement.

Metabolism & Excretion

Hepatic and renal

Adverse Reactions

Serious potential adverse reactions include closed-angle glaucoma, difficulty concentrating, hypokalemia, increased creatinine, kidney stones, metabolic acidosis, mood and sleep disorders, suicidal ideation, and tachycardia.

Side Effects

Constipation, dizziness, dry mouth, and paresthesia may occur.

Drug–Drug Interactions

Phentermine-topiramate may increase the risk of hypotension for individuals taking antihypertensives and hypoglycemia for individuals taking antidiabetic medications.

The concomitant use of alcohol or central nervous system (CNS) depressant drugs (such as barbiturates, benzodiazepines, hypnotics, and opioids) with phentermine-topiramate may potentiate CNS depression and dizziness, drowsiness, impaired concentration, and lightheadedness.

Concurrent use of phentermine-topiramate with non-potassium-sparing diuretics may potentiate the potassium-wasting action of these diuretics.

Concomitant administration of carbamazepine or phenytoin with topiramate for individuals with epilepsy may decrease the plasma concentrations of topiramate.

Concomitant use of topiramate with any other carbonic anhydrase inhibitor, such as acetazolamide, dichlorphenamide, or zonisamide, may increase the severity of metabolic acidosis and could increase the risk of kidney stone formation.

Specific Considerations for Women

Pregnancy

Phentermine-topiramate is contraindicated during pregnancy because weight loss is not recommended and could cause fetal harm. Additionally, data from pregnancy registries and epidemiology studies indicate that fetuses exposed to topiramate in the first trimester of pregnancy have an increased risk of oral clefts. Effective contraception should be used during treatment with phentermine-topiramate. If a woman becomes pregnant while taking phentermine-topiramate, the medication should be discontinued as soon as the pregnancy is recognized.

Breastfeeding

There is no information on combination use of phentermine-topiramate or phentermine alone during breastfeeding. Limited data suggest that topiramate is excreted in breast milk in small amounts. Medications to promote weight loss are generally not recommended during lactation.

Nonpharmacologic interventions, such as dietary and lifestyle modifications, are the first-line modalities for weight control while breastfeeding.

Adolescent women
There are no safety data on the use of phentermine-topiramate for women under age 18.

Elderly women
There are no data to suggest that individuals who are older respond differently from those who are younger. However, individuals who are older may be more sensitive to the CNS adverse effects of phentermine-topiramate. This medication is primarily excreted by the kidneys, and the risk of adverse reactions may be greater for individuals with impaired renal function, which is more common among the elderly.

Dose
Phentermine-topiramate is started at doses of 3.75 mg/23 mg taken orally each day for 14 days, then increased to 7.5 mg/46 mg daily. After 12 weeks, the dose is increased to 11.25 mg/69 mg if 3% weight loss is not achieved. After 2 weeks, the dose is increased to a maximum of 15 mg/92 mg. If 5% weight loss is not achieved after 12 weeks at this highest dose, the medication should be discontinued slowly, as continuing phentermine-topiramate is unlikely to be effective after dose escalations.

The 3.75-mg/23-mg and 11.25-mg/69-mg doses are for titration only.

Dose adjustments:
Moderate to severe renal impairment: maximum dose is 7.5 mg/46 mg orally once daily.

Moderate hepatic impairment: maximum dose is 7.5 mg/46 mg orally once daily.

How Supplied
Phentermine-topiramate is supplied as extended-release capsules for oral use containing phentermine/topiramate in the following strengths:
    3.75 mg/23 mg
    7.5 mg/46 mg
    11.25 mg/69 mg
    15 mg/92 mg

Prescribing Considerations

Topiramate may cause an increase in fetal oral clefts and should not be taken during pregnancy. A negative pregnancy test should be documented prior to beginning treatment with phentermine-topiramate and each month prior to renewing the prescription.

Phentermine-topiramate is available only through a Risk Evaluation and Mitigation Strategy (REMS) program. This program requires provider training and restricts access through pharmacies that are enrolled in the phentermine-topiramate (Qsymia) certified pharmacy network. The purpose of the REMS program is to inform healthcare providers and women of reproductive age about (1) the increased risk of congenital malformation, specifically orofacial clefts, for infants exposed to phentermine-topiramate during the first trimester of pregnancy; (2) the importance of pregnancy prevention for women of reproductive age receiving phentermine-topiramate; and (3) the need to discontinue phentermine-topiramate immediately if pregnancy occurs. Additional information may be obtained via the website (www.QsymiaREMS.com) or by telephone at 1-888-998-4887.

Phentermine-topiramate is a Schedule IV drug per the Controlled Substances Act because it contains phentermine, a Schedule IV drug, and has a known potential for abuse. It should be used with caution by individuals with a history of substance abuse.

Phentermine-topiramate should be taken in the morning to reduce the risk of insomnia that might occur with bedtime use.

To discontinue, one dose of phentermine-topiramate 15 mg/92 mg should be taken every other day for at least 1 week prior to stopping treatment altogether, to reduce the risk of precipitating a seizure.

Use with alcohol should be avoided.

Cost: $$$$$

Podofilox gel, 0.5% (Condylox)

Therapeutic class: Keratolytic

Chemical class: Antimitotic

Indications
Podofilox is indicated for the topical treatment of anogenital warts, including external genital warts (EGWs) and perianal warts. It is not indicated for the treatment of mucous membrane warts that appear on the rectum, urethra, or vagina.

Contraindications
Podofilox is contraindicated for individuals with a known allergy, hypersensitivity, or intolerance to any components of the medication or gel.

Mechanism of Action
Treatment with podofilox results in necrosis of visible wart tissue.

Metabolism & Excretion
Not applicable

Adverse Reactions
No serious adverse reactions are associated with podofilox use.

Side Effects
Common side effects are local skin reactions that may include bleeding, burning, erosion, inflammation, itching, and pain.

Drug–Drug Interactions
There are no known clinically significant drug–drug interactions.

Specific Considerations for Women
Pregnancy
Podofilox is an antimitotic drug, and these medications are known to be embryotoxic. However, topical application does not result in detectable serum levels. There are no adequate and well-controlled studies that have included women who are pregnant. The CDC STD Treatment Guidelines state that podofilox is not recommended during pregnancy. If EGWs proliferate and become friable, an alternate method of removal, such as freezing, should be considered.

Breastfeeding
There are no data on the use of podofilox during breastfeeding. Topical application of podofilox to external genitalia does not result in detectable

serum levels, and the drug does not accumulate after multiple treatments. There are no expected adverse effects for infants who are breastfeeding.

Adolescent women
Adolescent women may use podofilox.

Elderly women
Women who are postmenopausal and have EGWs may use podofilox; there are no data to suggest that women who are older respond differently than women who are younger. However, as women age, more fragile skin may be prone to injury and women with adverse skin reactions should be monitored closely.

Dose
Podofilox should be applied to EGWs with the applicator tip or finger. Application should be done twice daily for 3 consecutive days, then discontinued for 4 consecutive days. This one-week cycle of treatment may be repeated until there is no visible wart tissue or for a maximum of four cycles.

How Supplied
Podofilox gel 0.5% is supplied as 3.5 grams of clear gel in aluminum tubes with an applicator tip.

Prescribing Considerations
If there is no resolution of EGWs after four weeks of treatment, podofilox should be discontinued and another therapy considered. More frequent applications will increase the chance of adverse skin reactions.

The gel should be allowed to dry completely before the patient gets dressed and resumes normal activities.

Any gel that is on hands or fingers should be washed off thoroughly. Contact with the eyes should be avoided.

Sexual activity should be avoided during days podofilox is applied.

Podofilox can be used during a woman's menstrual cycle, but the gel should be dry before changing tampons or inserting/removing a menstrual cup to avoid inadvertent introduction of the gel into the vagina.

Vaccination with the 9-valent human papilloma virus vaccine should be considered as a routine measure.

Cost: $$$$$

Prasterone (Intrarosa)

Therapeutic class: Endocrine-metabolic agent

Chemical class: Synthetic steroid identical to naturally occurring pro-hormone 5-dehydroepiandrosterone (5-DHEA)

Indications
Prasterone is indicated for the treatment of moderate to severe dyspareunia secondary to vaginal and vulvar atrophy of menopause.

Contraindications
Prasterone is contraindicated for women with undiagnosed vaginal bleeding.
Prasterone is not indicated during pregnancy.

Mechanism of Action
Prasterone is an inactive endogenous steroid and is converted into active androgens and/or estrogens. The mechanism of action of prasterone for postmenopausal women with vaginal or vulvar atrophy is not fully established.

Metabolism & Excretion
Unknown

Adverse Reactions
Pap smear changes may occur with the use of prasterone, including ASCUS and LSIL.

Side Effects
Increased vaginal discharge can occur.

Drug–Drug Interactions
Estrogen is a metabolite of prasterone, and this medication has not been studied for women with a past or current history of breast cancer.

Specific Considerations for Women
Pregnancy
Prasterone is only indicated for women who are postmenopausal and should not be used by women who are pregnant. There are no data on prasterone

use during pregnancy, and drug-associated risks are unknown. Animal studies have not been conducted.

Breastfeeding
Prasterone is only indicated for women who are postmenopausal. There is no information on the presence of prasterone in human milk, the effects on an infant who is breastfeeding, or the effects on milk production. Women who are experiencing dyspareunia during breastfeeding should not use prasterone. Water-soluble vaginal lubricants may be an alternative for dyspareunia that is associated with breastfeeding.

Adolescent women
Adolescent women are not postmenopausal, and therefore prasterone is not indicated for this population.

Elderly women
No differences in safety or effectiveness have been noted between older and younger women who are postmenopausal. No dose adjustment is required for women over 65 years of age.

Dose
One insert is used vaginally each night at bedtime.

How Supplied
Supplied as a vaginal insert containing 6.5 mg of prasterone. One box contains 28 inserts and applicators.

Prescribing Considerations
It may take up to 12 weeks for women to notice improvement in symptoms.

There are no restrictions on length of use. Women should be assessed for improvement in symptoms and decisions on duration of treatment made on an individual basis.

Women using prasterone should continue routine Pap smear screening based on national guidelines.

Abnormal bleeding during treatment should be investigated clinically.

Cost: $$$$$

Pregabalin (Lyrica)

Therapeutic class: Neuropathic pain agent

Chemical class: Anticonvulsant

Indications
Pregabalin is indicated for the treatment of:

1. Neuropathic pain associated with diabetic peripheral neuropathy (DPN)
2. Postherpetic neuralgia (PHN)
3. Adjunctive therapy for adults with partial-onset seizures
4. Fibromyalgia

Contraindications
Pregabalin is contraindicated for individuals with known hypersensitivity to pregabalin or any of its components.

Mechanism of Action
Pregabalin binds to the alpha 2-delta site in central nervous system (CNS) tissues. This binding may be involved in antinociceptive and antiseizure effects. The antinociceptive activities of pregabalin may also be mediated through interactions with descending noradrenergic and serotonergic pathways that modulate pain transmission in the spinal cord.

Metabolism & Excretion
Negligible hepatic metabolism, excreted renally

Adverse Reactions
Potentially serious adverse reactions are possible and include angioedema, creatine kinase elevations resulting in muscle pain and weakness, hypersensitivity reactions, mood changes, reduction in platelet count, skin ulcers, and suicidal thoughts.

Side Effects
Blurred vision, dizziness, dry mouth, edema, somnolence, weight gain

Drug–Drug Interactions

Taking pregabalin with other CNS depressants, such as alcohol, benzodiazepines, and opioids, will increase the risk of dizziness, drowsiness, and somnolence.

Specific Considerations for Women

Pregnancy

There are no well-controlled studies of pregabalin use by women who are pregnant, although animal studies have suggested structural abnormalities and growth restriction. The clinical need for the medication should be weighed against possible risks. Healthcare providers are advised to encourage women who are pregnant and taking pregabalin to enroll in the North American Antiepileptic Drug (NAAED) Pregnancy Registry. This can be done by calling 1-888-233-2334 and must be done by women themselves. Registry information can also be found at http://www.aedpregnancyregistry.org/.

Breastfeeding

There are limited data on pregabalin and breastfeeding, but levels in breast milk appear to be low. Women can breastfeed older infants while taking pregabalin but should be cautious with neonates, who are expected to receive more medication via breast milk.

Adolescent women

The safety and efficacy of pregabalin have not been established for individuals under age 18.

Elderly women

No differences in safety or effectiveness have been noted between older and younger women. There are no recommended age-related dose reductions.

Dose: Variable, depending on the condition being treated

Adjunct therapy for partial-onset seizures:

Initial dose is 75 mg orally two times per day, or 50 mg three times per day. The dose may be increased to a maximum daily dose of 600 mg.

Fibromyalgia:
Initial dose is 75 mg orally two times per day. The dose may be increased to 150 mg two times per day (300 mg per day). If adequate benefit is not achieved, the dose may be further increased to 225 mg two times per day, for a maximum daily dose of 450 mg.

Neuropathic pain associated with diabetic neuropathy:
Initial dose is 50 mg orally three times per day. May be increased to 100 mg three times per day for a maximum of 300 mg daily.

Postherpetic neuralgia:
Initial dose is 75 mg orally two times per day, or 50 mg three times per day. May be increased to 100 mg three times per day (300 mg daily). If adequate pain relief is not achieved, the dose may be increased to 300 mg two times per day, or 200 mg three times per day, for a maximum daily dose of 600 mg.

Dose reductions are required for individuals with renal impairment. Refer to full prescribing information for suggested dose adjustments.

How Supplied
Pregabalin is supplied as 25-mg, 50-mg, 75-mg, 100-mg, 150-mg, 200-mg, 225-mg, and 300-mg capsules for oral use.

Prescribing Considerations
Pregabalin is a Schedule V controlled substance. Some individuals have reported euphoric effects while taking pregabalin. History of substance abuse should be assessed prior to beginning treatment.

Changes in mood or suicidal thoughts should be reported to a healthcare provider immediately.

Abrupt discontinuation may result in diarrhea, headache, insomnia, and nausea. The dose should be gradually reduced over the course of one week to reduce the risk of withdrawal symptoms.

Alcohol use should be avoided or greatly reduced while taking pregabalin.

Activities that require mental alertness, such as driving, should be avoided until effects of pregabalin are known.

Individuals with reduced renal function will need lower doses of pregabalin.

Cost: $$$$$

Progesterone intrauterine devices (IUDs) (Kyleena, Liletta, Mirena, Skyla)

Therapeutic class: Contraceptive

Chemical class: Progestin

Indications
Long-acting contraception for the prevention of pregnancy.

The Mirena IUD also has an indication for the treatment of heavy menstrual bleeding.

The 52-mg progestin IUDs have been used off label for endometrial protection during perimenopausal estrogen treatment, to reduce abnormal bleeding of perimenopause, and for menstrual suppression.

Contraindications
In general, progestin IUDs are contraindicated with the following conditions:

1. Pregnancy or suspected pregnancy
2. Congenital or acquired uterine anomaly, including fibroids if they distort the uterine cavity
3. Acute pelvic inflammatory disease (PID) or a history of PID, unless there has been a subsequent intrauterine pregnancy
4. Postpartum endometritis or infected abortion in the past 3 months
5. Known or suspected uterine or cervical neoplasia or unresolved, abnormal Pap smear
6. Vaginal bleeding of unknown etiology
7. Untreated acute cervicitis or vaginitis, including bacterial vaginosis or other lower genital tract infections, until infection is treated
8. Acute liver disease or liver tumor (benign or malignant)

P

9. Conditions associated with increased susceptibility to pelvic infections
10. A previously inserted IUD that has not been removed
11. Hypersensitivity to any component of the product
12. Known or suspected carcinoma of the breast

Mechanism of Action
Prevention of pregnancy occurs through several mechanisms, including thickening of cervical mucus that blocks passage of sperm into the uterus, inhibition of sperm capacitation or survival, and alteration of the endometrium.

Metabolism & Excretion
Hepatic and renal; minimal systemic absorption

Adverse Reactions
Although the risk of pregnancy is low, if a pregnancy does occur with a progestin IUD, there is a greater risk of an ectopic pregnancy.

Sepsis and PID are possible. Embedment, expulsion, and perforation have occurred.

Ovulation may not be suppressed with progestin IUDs, and ovarian cysts can develop.

Side Effects
Progestin IUDs will alter the menstrual bleeding pattern and may result in irregular and unscheduled bleeding or induce amenorrhea. Other possible side effects include abdominal cramping, acne, breast tenderness, headache, and vaginal discharge.

Drug–Drug Interactions
There are no known clinically significant drug–drug interactions.

Specific Considerations for Women
Pregnancy
Progestin IUDs are contraindicated during pregnancy. If a pregnancy is diagnosed with an IUD in place, the IUD should be removed to decrease the chance of sepsis. IUD removal may lead to pregnancy loss.

Breastfeeding
Woman may use progestin IUDs while breastfeeding.

Adolescent women
Progestin IUDs may be used by adolescent women.

Elderly women
Women who are postmenopausal do not have a menstrual cycle or require contraception.

Dose
Kyleena: 19.5 mg of levonorgestrel, 5 years of use
  Liletta: 52 mg of levonorgestrel, 5 years of use (evidence-based for 7 years)
  Mirena: 52 mg of levonorgestrel, 5 years of use (evidence-based for 7 years)
  Skyla: 13.5 mg of levonorgestrel, 3 years of use

How Supplied
Each progestin IUD is supplied as a single unit for individual use.

Prescribing Considerations
The different progestin IUDs each require slightly different insertion techniques. Providers should receive specific training on the IUD they are inserting. Detailed instructions are included with the package labeling.

Progestin IUDs can be placed at any time during the menstrual cycle if the provider is reasonably certain the woman is not pregnant. Documenting a negative pregnancy test prior to insertion is prudent.

Nucleic acid amplification testing (NAAT) for chlamydia and gonorrhea should be obtained at insertion if women have not had routine screening or if they have risk factors for sexually transmitted infections (STIs) based on their history. Infections should be treated appropriately, but insertion should not be delayed while waiting for test results. The greatest risk for PID is within the first 21 days after insertion if there is an active cervical infection.

Consider offering a follow-up appointment approximately 6 weeks after insertion to assess any concerns. Although this visit is not medically necessary, it does allow for a discussion of any bothersome side effects, including changes in the menstrual cycle. However, women can decide individually if they are interested in a postinsertion visit.

The IUD should be removed or changed after the appropriate time, depending on the device used.

Review possible adverse reactions, including expected changes in bleeding pattern.

Progestin IUDs do not protect against STIs or HIV.

Cost: $$$$$

Progesterone micronized (Prometrium)

Therapeutic class: Hormone/hormone replacement

Chemical class: Progestin

Indications
Micronized progesterone is indicated for use in the prevention of endometrial hyperplasia for women who are postmenopausal, have an intact uterus, and are receiving conjugated estrogens. Micronized progesterone is also indicated for the treatment of secondary amenorrhea.

Contraindications
Micronized progesterone is contraindicated with:

1. Known hypersensitivity to its ingredients. Prometrium capsules contain peanut oil and should never be used by women allergic to peanuts
2. Undiagnosed abnormal vaginal bleeding
3. Known, suspected, or history of breast cancer
4. Active deep vein thrombosis (DVT), pulmonary embolism (PE), or history of these conditions
5. Active arterial thromboembolic disease (cerebral vascular accident [CVA] or myocardial infarction [MI]) or a history of these conditions
6. Known liver dysfunction or disease
7. Known or suspected pregnancy

Mechanism of Action
Progesterone administration decreases the circulatory levels of gonadotropins. Progesterone can be used to achieve normalized progesterone levels for women with secondary amenorrhea.

Metabolism & Excretion
Hepatic and biliary

Adverse Reactions
Many of the reported adverse reactions have occurred during daily use of oral estrogen plus progesterone in the form of medroxyprogesterone acetate. It is unclear if the same risks exist for intermittent use of micronized progesterone only.

Potential adverse reactions include abnormal vaginal bleeding; breast, endometrial, and ovarian cancers; cardiovascular disorders; dementia; depression; elevated blood pressure and lipids; hepatic impairment; and visual changes.

Side Effects
Abdominal pain, acne, bloating, breast tenderness, fatigue, hair loss, headache, weight gain

Drug–Drug Interactions
Inhibitors of CYP450 3A4 may increase the bioavailability of progesterone. Specific drug–drug interaction studies evaluating the clinical effects with CYP450 3A4 inducers or inhibitors on micronized progesterone have not been conducted. However, inducers and/or inhibitors of CYP450 3A4 may affect the metabolism of progesterone.

Specific Considerations for Women
Pregnancy
Micronized progesterone is contraindicated during pregnancy. The conditions it is used for do not occur during pregnancy, and therefore it provides no therapeutic benefit for women who are pregnant. However, there do not appear to be any adverse effects for fetuses inadvertently exposed to micronized progesterone during the first trimester.

Breastfeeding
Oral progesterone is excreted in breast milk. Most information on lactation is the result of research on the depot medroxyprogesterone acetate (DMPA) contraceptive injection. DMPA has not been found to adversely affect the composition of milk, the growth and development of the infant, or the milk supply.

Adolescent women
Micronized progesterone has not been well studied with the pediatric population. Irregular menses and secondary amenorrhea are common among adolescents. All options to treat these conditions should be considered.

Elderly women
No differences in safety or effectiveness have been noted between older and younger women. There may be an increased risk of dementia for women over age 65 years when micronized progesterone is used with estrogen.

Dose
Prevention of endometrial hyperplasia:
A single 200-mg dose is taken orally at bedtime for 12 days sequentially per 28-day cycle, for women who are postmenopausal, have an intact uterus, and are taking daily conjugated estrogen tablets.

Treatment of secondary amenorrhea:
A single 400-mg dose is taken orally at bedtime for 10 days.

How Supplied
Micronized progesterone is supplied as 100-mg and 200-mg capsules for oral use.

Prescribing Considerations
Micronized progesterone has a **black box warning** for the possibility of breast cancer, cardiovascular events, and dementia when used with estrogen. However, this risk is based on data from use with combined estrogen and progesterone in the form of medroxyprogesterone acetate. It is unclear if the same risks exist for the intermittent use of micronized progesterone only.

Micronized progesterone (Prometrium) contains peanut oil. A careful allergy history should be obtained.

Abnormal vaginal bleeding should be reported to a healthcare provider and investigated appropriately.

Micronized progesterone may have a sedating effect and should be taken at bedtime.

The lowest dose for the shortest amount of time is prudent.

Cost: $–$$

Progesterone-only pills (Camila, Errin, Jolivette, Micronor, Nora-BE, Nor-QD)

Therapeutic class: Contraceptive

Chemical class: Progestin

Indications
Progestin-only pills (POPs) are indicated for the prevention of pregnancy.

Contraindications
POPs should not be used by women with:

1. Known or suspected pregnancy
2. Known or suspected carcinoma of the breast
3. Undiagnosed abnormal vaginal bleeding
4. Hypersensitivity to any component of the product
5. Benign or malignant liver tumors
6. Acute liver disease

Mechanism of Action
POPs prevent pregnancy through a variety of mechanisms, including suppressing ovulation for approximately half of users, thickening the cervical mucus to inhibit sperm penetration, lowering the midcycle luteinizing hormone (LH) and follicle stimulation hormone (FSH) peaks, slowing fallopian tube ovum transport, and altering the endometrium.

Metabolism & Excretion
Gastrointestinal (fecal), hepatic, and renal

Adverse Reactions
Adverse reactions that are possible with POPs include ectopic pregnancy, minor alterations in carbohydrate metabolism, and ovarian cysts.

Side Effects
Acne, alterations in the menstrual cycle, breast tenderness, headache, irregular vaginal bleeding, nausea, and spotting have been reported.

Drug–Drug Interactions
Hepatic enzyme-inducing drugs such as barbiturates, carbamazepine, phenytoin, and rifampin may reduce the effectiveness of POPs.

Specific Considerations for Women
Pregnancy
POPs are contraindicated during pregnancy because they provide no therapeutic benefit. However, no adverse outcomes have occurred for fetuses exposed to POPs.

Breastfeeding
Women who are breastfeeding may use POPs for contraception. According to U.S. Medical Eligibility Criteria for Contraceptive Use, POPs are a level 1 (more than 1 month postpartum) or level 2 (less than 1 month postpartum) recommendation.

Adolescent women
Adolescent women may use POPs.

Elderly women
Women who are postmenopausal are not at risk for pregnancy, and therefore POPs provide no therapeutic benefit.

Dose
POPs contain 0.35 mg norethindrone in each pill.

How Supplied
POPs are supplied as a single pack of 28 pills for oral use.

Prescribing Considerations

POPs do not provide protection against sexually transmitted infections (STIs) or HIV.

Pills should be taken daily at the same time, even during episodes of bleeding.

Late or missed pills increase the risk for unintended pregnancy.

Starting POPs on the first day of the menstrual cycle may decrease irregular bleeding.

Cost: $

Propranolol (Inderal)

Therapeutic class: Antihypertensive

Chemical class: Beta blocker. Other medications in this category include carvedilol, labetalol, and metoprolol.

Indications

Propranolol is indicated for the treatment and management of:

1. Hypertension
2. Angina pectoris due to coronary atherosclerosis
3. Atrial fibrillation
4. Myocardial infarction (MI)
5. Migraine prophylaxis
6. Essential tremor
7. Hypertrophic subaortic stenosis
8. Pheochromocytoma

P

Contraindications

Propranolol is contraindicated with:

1. Cardiogenic shock
2. Sinus bradycardia and greater than first-degree block
3. Bronchial asthma
4. Known hypersensitivity to propranolol hydrochloride

Mechanism of Action

Propranolol competes with beta-adrenergic receptor agonist agents for available receptor sites. When these sites are blocked, the chronotropic, inotropic, and vasodilator responses to beta-adrenergic stimulation are decreased. Antihypertensive effects may be related to decreased cardiac output, inhibition of renin release by the kidneys, and reduction of tonic sympathetic nerve outflow from vasomotor centers in the brain.

The mechanism of the antimigraine effect of propranolol has not been established, although beta adrenergic receptors are present in the pial vessels of the brain.

Metabolism & Excretion

Hepatic and renal

Adverse Reactions

Serious adverse reactions can include bradycardia in the presence of Wolf-Parkinson-White syndrome, cardiac failure, hyperthyroidism, masking of symptoms of hypoglycemia, nonallergic bronchospasm, severe hypersensitivity reactions, and worsening of angina or MI with abrupt discontinuation.

Side Effects

Dizziness, fatigue, insomnia, lethargy, lightheadedness, nausea, rash, reduced intraocular pressure, weakness

Drug–Drug Interactions

The metabolism of propranolol involves multiple pathways in the cytochrome P-450 system.

Propranolol levels may be increased by co-administration with substrates or inhibitors of CYP2D6 (amiodarone, cimetidine, delavudin, fluoxetine, paroxetine, quinidine, ritonavir), substrates or inhibitors of CYP1A2 (ciprofloxacin, fluvoxamine, imipramine, isoniazid, rizatriptan, theophylline, zileuton, zolmitriptan), and substrates or inhibitors of CYP2C19 (fluconazole, teniposide, tolbutamide).

Propranolol levels may be decreased by co-administration with inducers such as ethanol, phenytoin, phenobarbital, and rifampin.

Cigarette smoking induces hepatic metabolism and has been shown to increase the clearance of propranolol, resulting in decreased plasma concentrations.

Many other drug–drug interactions are possible. Consult full prescribing information prior to initiating treatment with propranolol.

Specific Considerations for Women
Pregnancy
There are no adequate and well-controlled studies of propranolol use by women who are pregnant. Beta blockers may cause decreased placental perfusion, fetal and neonatal bradycardia and hypoglycemia, intrauterine growth restriction, and small placentas. Propranolol should only be used if there is no adequate alternative and the potential benefit justifies the potential risk to the fetus. Labetalol may be an alternative medication during pregnancy.

Breastfeeding
Propranolol is excreted in breast milk in low amounts. There have been recognized adverse effects for infants who are breastfeeding. Other medications should be considered.

Adolescent women
Per package labeling, safety and efficacy have not been established for individuals under age 18.

Elderly women
No differences in safety or effectiveness have been noted between older and younger women. Other comorbid conditions or medications may increase the risk of adverse effects. Using the lowest effective dose may reduce the risk of adverse reactions.

Dose: Variable, depending on condition being treated
Angina pectoris:
Total daily doses range from 80 mg to 320 mg orally, two, three, or four times per day.

Atrial fibrillation:
The recommended dose is 10 mg to 30 mg orally three or four times daily before meals and at bedtime.

Essential tremor:
The initial dose is 40 mg orally twice daily. Optimum reduction of essential tremor is usually achieved with a total dose of 120 mg per day.

Hypertension:
The usual initial dose is 40 mg orally twice daily. The usual maintenance dose is 120 mg to 240 mg per day.

Hypertrophic subaortic stenosis:
The usual dose is 20 mg to 40 mg orally three or four times daily before meals and at bedtime.

MI:
The usual initial dose is 40 mg orally three or four times per day, with titration after 1 month to 60 mg to 80 mg orally three to four times per day as tolerated. The recommended daily maintenance dose is 180 mg to 240 mg orally in divided doses.

Migraine:
The initial dose is 80 mg orally daily in divided doses. The usual effective dose range is 160 mg to 240 mg per day. If a satisfactory reduction in migraine headaches is not obtained within 4 to 6 weeks after reaching the maximum dose, treatment with propranolol should be discontinued gradually over a period of several weeks.

Pheochromocytoma:
The usual dosage is 60 mg orally daily in divided doses for 3 days prior to surgery. For management of inoperable tumors, the usual dose is 30 mg orally daily in divided doses as adjunctive therapy to alpha-adrenergic blockade.

How Supplied
Propranolol is supplied as tablets for oral use in doses of 10 mg, 20 mg, 40 mg, 60 mg, and 80 mg.

Prescribing Considerations

Propranolol is used for migraine prophylaxis and will not improve a migraine in progress.

A slow discontinuation of propranolol should occur over the course of a few weeks.

Multiple medication interactions are possible. A complete medication history should be taken prior to initiating treatment with propranolol.

Alternate beta-blockers exist that can have different indications, doses, and prices. Choice of medication should be individualized to the specific needs of each woman.

Cost: $–$$

Raloxifene (Evista)

Therapeutic class: Antineoplastic; anti-osteoporotic

Chemical class: Estrogen agonist/antagonist; selective estrogen receptor modulator (SERM)

Indications

Raloxifene is indicated for the:

1. Treatment and prevention of osteoporosis for women who are postmenopausal
2. Reduction in risk of invasive breast cancer for women with osteoporosis who are postmenopausal
3. Reduction in risk of invasive breast cancer for women who are post-menopausal and at high risk for invasive breast cancer

Contraindications

Women with current or past stroke or venous thromboembolism (VTE) (including deep vein thrombosis [DVT], pulmonary embolism [PE], and retinal vein thrombosis) should not take raloxifene.

Raloxifene is contraindicated during pregnancy.

R

Mechanism of Action
Raloxifene binds estrogen receptors, which results in activation of estrogenic pathways in some tissues (agonism) and blockade of estrogenic pathways in others (antagonism). Raloxifene acts as an estrogen agonist in bone, decreases bone resorption and bone turnover, increases bone mineral density (BMD), and decreases fracture incidence.

Metabolism & Excretion
Renal and gastrointestinal (fecal)

Adverse Reactions
DVT, PE, stroke, VTE (see Contraindications)

May increase triglycerides for women with marked hypertriglyceridemia (more than 500 mg/dL).

Side Effects
The most commonly reported side effects are arthralgia, edema, flu-like symptoms, hot flashes/hot flushes, leg cramps, and sweating.

Drug–Drug Interactions
Raloxifene should not be administered concurrently with estrogen.

Cholestyramine decreases raloxifene levels.

Raloxifene may interact with warfarin, and women taking both medications should have prothrombin time monitored closely.

Specific Considerations for Women
Pregnancy
Raloxifene is contraindicated during pregnancy and may cause fetal harm. It is only indicated for postmenopausal use.

Breastfeeding
It is not known if raloxifene is excreted in breast milk. It is only indicated for postmenopausal use and should not be prescribed to women who are breastfeeding.

Adolescent women
Raloxifene is indicated for women who are postmenopausal and is not appropriate for the adolescent population.

Elderly women

No differences in safety or effectiveness have been noted between older and younger women who are postmenopausal. A dose adjustment is not indicated for women who are elderly (over age 65).

Dose

One 60-mg tablet orally daily.

How Supplied

Raloxifene is supplied as a 60-mg tablet for oral use.

Prescribing Considerations

Raloxifene has a **black box warning** for the increased risk of VTE and death and should not be taken by women with a history of VTE events.

Raloxifene should be discontinued at least 72 hours prior to and during prolonged immobilization, and women should be advised to avoid prolonged restrictions of movement during travel due to the increased risk of VTE events.

Raloxifene does not eliminate the risk of breast cancer. Women should have a clinical breast exam and mammogram prior to starting raloxifene and continue with regular breast exams and mammograms during treatment, per national guidelines.

If raloxifene is given for the prevention or treatment of osteoporosis, supplemental calcium and/or vitamin D should be considered if dietary intake is inadequate.

Raloxifene should not be given for the primary or secondary prevention of heart disease.

Any unexplained vaginal bleeding that occurs during raloxifene treatment should be investigated clinically.

Raloxifene may increase the incidence of hot flashes and flushes.

Lipids should be monitored during treatment with raloxifene.

Cost: $$

Secnidazole (Solosec)

Therapeutic class: Antibiotic and antiprotozoal

Chemical class: Nitroimidazole derivative. Other medications in this category include metronidazole and tinidazole.

Indications
Secnidazole is indicated for adult women in the treatment of bacterial vaginosis (BV).

Contraindications
Secnidazole is contraindicated for individuals with a known hypersensitivity to the medication, other ingredients of the formulation, or other nitroimidazole derivatives.

Mechanism of Action
Secnidazole is a 5-nitroimidazole antimicrobial that enters the bacterial cell and results in nitro group reduction by bacterial enzymes to radical anions. It is believed that these radical anions interfere with bacterial DNA synthesis of susceptible isolates.

Metabolism & Excretion
Hepatic and renal

Adverse Reactions
Carcinogenicity has been reported in mice and rats treated chronically with nitroimidazole derivatives that are structurally related to secnidazole. It is unclear how carcinogenicity seen with other nitroimidazole derivatives in animals relates to a single dose of secnidazole in humans.

Side Effects
The most common side effect is vulvovaginal candidiasis. Abdominal pain, diarrhea, headache, nausea, and vomiting may occur.

Drug–Drug Interactions
There are no known clinically significant drug–drug interactions.

Specific Considerations for Women
Pregnancy
There are no adequate and well-controlled studies of secnidazole use among women who are pregnant. According to the CDC STD Treatment Guidelines, women with symptomatic BV who are pregnant should be treated with either oral or vaginal metronidazole preparations.

Breastfeeding
No information is available on the clinical use of secnidazole during breast-feeding or the effects on the infant who is breastfeeding. It is presumed that potential adverse effects are similar to those of metronidazole, which is a closely related drug. Maternal ingestion of oral metronidazole may increase the risk of oral and rectal *Candida* infections for the infant. As with metronidazole, concern has been raised about exposure of healthy infants to secnidazole via breast milk because of possible mutagenicity and carcinogenicity. Product labeling recommends avoidance of breastfeeding for 96 hours after a single dose. Other drugs are available for the treatment of BV, including vaginal metronidazole, which should result in lower amounts in breast milk.

Adolescent women
The safety and efficacy of secnidazole have not been established for women under age 18.

Elderly women
No differences in safety or effectiveness have been noted between older and younger women.

Dose
Secnidazole is given orally as a 2-gram single dose.

How Supplied
Secnidazole is available as a single packet containing 2 grams in oral granules.

Prescribing Considerations
The entire packet of secnidazole granules should be sprinkled on apple-sauce, pudding, or yogurt and consumed within 30 minutes without

chewing or crunching the granules. A glass of water can be used to help with swallowing, but secnidazole should not be dissolved in water or any other liquid.

Secnidazole may be an option for treatment of BV for women who have difficulty swallowing pills and do not want to use a vaginal preparation.

Other nitroimidazole medications, such as metronidazole and tinidazole, are available that may have a different dosing schedule and cost. Choice of medication should be individualized to the specific needs of each woman.

Cost: $$$$–$$$$$

Sertraline (Zoloft)

Therapeutic class: Antidepressant

Chemical class: Selective serotonin reuptake inhibitor (SSRI). Other medications in this category include citalopram, escitalopram, fluoxetine, paroxetine, and vilazodone.

Indications
Sertraline is indicated for the treatment of:

1. Major depressive disorder (MDD)
2. Obsessive-compulsive disorder (OCD)
3. Panic disorder
4. Post-traumatic stress disorder (PTSD)
5. Social anxiety disorder
6. Premenstrual dysphoric disorder (PMDD)

Contraindications
Sertraline is contraindicated with the use of monoamine oxidase inhibitors (MAOIs) or use within 14 days of stopping MAOIs. Sertraline is also contraindicated with the use of pimozide.

Sertraline is contraindicated with known hypersensitivity to sertraline or other SSRIs.

Mechanism of Action
Sertraline potentiates serotonergic activity in the central nervous system (CNS) through inhibition of neuronal reuptake of serotonin (5-HT).

Metabolism & Excretion
Hepatic and gastrointestinal (fecal)

Adverse Reactions
Significant adverse reactions include the possibility of closed-angle glaucoma, hyponatremia, increased risk of bleeding, mania, mood changes and suicidality, QTc prolongation, seizures, and serotonin syndrome.

Side Effects
Agitation, constipation, decreased libido, diarrhea, dizziness, dry mouth, fatigue, nausea, somnolence

Drug–Drug Interactions
Sertraline has significant interactions with MAOIs and pimozide (see Contraindications).

The risk of serotonin syndrome is increased when SSRIs, including sertraline, are taken with other serotonergic drugs such as amphetamines, buspirone, fentanyl, lithium, St. John's wort, tramadol, tricyclic antidepressants (TCAs), triptans, and tryptophan.

Use of sertraline with anti-platelet drugs, aspirin, nonsteroidal anti-inflammatory drugs (NSAIDs), other anticoagulants, and warfarin may increase the risk for bleeding.

Sertraline is a CYP2D6 inhibitor. It may increase the exposure of the CYP2D6 substrate.

Specific Considerations for Women
Pregnancy
Overall, there does not appear to be an increase in congenital malformations above the background rate for birth defects for infants exposed to sertraline during the first trimester. Infants exposed to SSRIs, including sertraline, during the third trimester can exhibit withdrawal symptoms after birth, including irritability, persistent pulmonary hypertension of the newborn

(PPHN), and prolonged hospitalization. Untreated maternal depression during pregnancy carries risks to the fetus. Need for the medication should be evaluated to balance risks of maternal depression with potential risks for the fetus.

Breastfeeding
Sertraline is present in low levels in breast milk. Sertraline is a preferred SSRI for women who are breastfeeding.

Adolescent women
Adolescent women may take sertraline. Adolescents who take sertraline should be closely monitored for changes in mood and suicidal thoughts and behaviors.

Elderly women
No differences in safety and effectiveness have been observed between older and younger individuals. Dosing should begin at the low end of the therapeutic dose range for individuals over age 65.

Dose: Variable, depending on condition being treated
MDD:
50 mg orally once daily

OCD:
50 mg orally once daily

Panic disorder:
25 mg orally once daily

PMDD:
50 mg orally once daily. Can be given every day of the menstrual cycle or intermittently starting 14 days prior to the anticipated onset of menses (luteal phase). With continuous dosing for PMDD, sertraline may be increased to a maximum of 150 mg daily. With intermittent dosing, sertraline can be given as 50 mg daily for the first 3 days of the luteal phase and then increased to 100 mg daily until menses begin.

PTSD:
25 mg orally once daily. The usual therapeutic range is 50 mg to 200 mg daily.

Social anxiety disorder:
25 mg orally once daily

How Supplied
Sertraline is supplied as 25-mg, 50-mg, and 100-mg tablets for oral use.

Prescribing Considerations
Sertraline has a **black box warning** for an increased risk of suicidality for children, adolescents, and young adults. Adolescents taking sertraline should be monitored closely and advised to report any changes in mood or new or worsening psychiatric symptoms.

Withdrawal symptoms can occur with abrupt discontinuation of sertraline. Individuals should be tapered off sertraline gradually.

Prior to initiating treatment with an antidepressant, individuals should be screened for bipolar disorder to reduce the risk of inducing a mixed/manic episode.

Sertraline should not be taken concurrently with an MAOI. A 14-day period should occur after stopping an MAOI before beginning sertraline, and an MAOI shouldn't be started until 14 days after stopping sertraline.

Sertraline may cause a false positive urine immunoassay for benzodiazepines.

Other SSRIs are available that may have a different dosing schedule and cost. Choice of medication should be individualized to the specific needs of each woman.

Cost: $–$$

Sinecatechins 15% ointment (Veregen)

S

Therapeutic class: Keratolytic

Chemical class: Botanical

Indications
Sinecatechins is a botanical product containing extracts from green tea leaves, primarily catechins and other green tea extracts. As an ointment,

it is indicated for the topical treatment of external genital warts (EGWs), including perianal warts (*Condylomata acuminata*) for individuals 18 years and older who are not immunocompromised.

Contraindications
Sinecatechins ointment is contraindicated if there is a history of hypersensitivity to the components in the medication. It should not be used on open wounds or skin that is not intact. Safety has not been established for individuals who are immunocompromised.

Mechanism of Action
The mode of action of sinecatechins ointment for the clearance of EGWs is unknown. In vitro, sinecatechins shows antioxidative activity, but it is unknown if this is the only mechanism involved in eradication of EGWs. Systemically administered green tea extracts have demonstrated antioxidant activity, but whether this applies to sinecatechins ointment is unclear.

Metabolism & Excretion
Not applicable

Adverse Reactions
No serious adverse reactions have been associated with the use of sinecatechins ointment.

Side Effects
The most common side effects are local skin reactions, including blisters, burning, erythema, itching, pain, and swelling. These reactions are experienced to some extent by most individuals during treatment.

Drug–Drug Interactions
There are no known clinically significant drug–drug interactions.

Specific Considerations for Women
Pregnancy
There are no adequate and well-controlled studies of sinecatechins ointment use among women who are pregnant. All available treatment options for EGWs during pregnancy should be considered and the potential benefit

of sinecatechins should be weighed against any potential unknown risks. Treatment of EGWs during pregnancy is not essential and unless the EGWs are large, friable, or causing significant discomfort, treatment can often be delayed until after delivery.

Breastfeeding
It is not known if the major components of sinecatechins ointment (catechins) are excreted in breast milk. The ointment is a water extract of green tea leaves that is thought to be safe during breastfeeding when consumed in moderation. There are no published studies examining topical sinecatechins applied to EGWs during breastfeeding. Topical products applied away from the breast should pose a negligible risk for the infant who is breastfeeding, but confirmatory data are lacking.

Adolescent women
Sinecatechins ointment may be used by adolescent women.

Elderly women
There is no evidence to indicate that women who are older respond differently than women who are younger. As women age, the skin may be more fragile and prone to injury. Adverse skin reactions should be monitored closely.

Dose
A thin layer of sinecatechins ointment should be applied with the fingertip to cover each EGW. The ointment is applied three times per day, typically on a morning, noon, and nighttime schedule. The previous application should not be washed off prior to the next. The duration of treatment is a maximum of 16 weeks.

How Supplied
Sinecatechins 15% ointment is supplied in aluminum tubes containing 15 grams of ointment per tube.

Prescribing Considerations
Sexual activity (anal, oral, vaginal) should be avoided when sinecatechins ointment is on the skin, or the ointment should be washed off prior to sex.

The ointment may weaken latex condoms or diaphragms and should not come in contact with latex barrier methods of contraception.

The ointment is brown and may stain light-colored clothing and bedding. Women should consider wearing darker-colored undergarments during treatment.

Local skin reactions occur frequently. Treatment should be continued unless there is significant discomfort or skin breakdown. Reports of major skin reactions should be evaluated clinically, at which time a decision can be made about continuing treatment.

Women who are using tampons or a menstrual cup during treatment with sinecatechins ointment should apply the ointment after the tampon or menstrual cup has been inserted. When changing tampons or emptying/reinserting a menstrual cup after the ointment has been applied, women should be careful not to introduce the ointment accidently into the vagina.

It is not known whether treatment with sinecatechins ointment reduces the risk of transmission of EGWs.

Vaccination with the 9-valent human papilloma virus vaccine should be considered as a routine measure.

Cost: $$$$$

Solifenacin (VESIcare)

Therapeutic class: Urinary antispasmodic

Chemical class: Bladder-selective muscarinic antagonist. Other medications in this category include darifenacin, oxybutynin, and tolterodine.

Indications
Solifenacin is indicated for the treatment of overactive bladder (OAB) with symptoms of urge urinary incontinence, urgency, and urinary frequency.

Contraindications
Solifenacin is contraindicated for individuals with:

1. Urinary or gastric retention

2. Uncontrolled narrow-angle glaucoma
3. Demonstrated hypersensitivity to the drug

Mechanism of Action
Solifenacin is a competitive muscarinic receptor antagonist. Muscarinic receptors play an important role in several cholinergically mediated functions, including contractions of urinary bladder smooth muscle.

Metabolism & Excretion
Hepatic and renal

Adverse Reactions
Potentially serious adverse reactions include angioedema and anaphylaxis, central nervous system (CNS) anticholinergic effects (confusion, hallucinations, headache, somnolence), increased QT prolongation, urinary retention, and severe constipation.

Side Effects
Abdominal pain, blurry vision, constipation, dry mouth, nausea

Drug–Drug Interactions
Inhibitors of CYP3A4 may increase the concentration of solifenacin, and inducers of CYP3A4 may decrease the concentration of solifenacin.

Specific Considerations for Women
Pregnancy
There are no adequate, well-controlled studies of solifenacin use by women who are pregnant. Medications for OAB are generally not prescribed during pregnancy.

Breastfeeding
There are no published data on use of solifenacin among women who are breastfeeding. It is not known if solifenacin is excreted in breast milk. However, if excreted, the drug has a long half-life (approximately 55 hours), which increases the possibility of infant exposure from breast milk.

Adolescent women
Safety and efficacy have not been established for women under age 18.

Elderly women

No differences in safety or effectiveness have been noted between older and younger women.

Dose

The recommended dose of solifenacin is 5 mg orally once daily. If the 5-mg dose is well tolerated but symptoms are not adequately controlled, the dose may be increased to 10 mg once daily.

Dose adjustments:

The daily dose should not exceed 5 mg for individuals with severe renal impairment (creatinine clearance less than 30 ml/min) or for individuals with moderate hepatic impairment.

The daily dose of solifenacin also should not exceed 5 mg daily for individuals who are also taking a potent CYP3A4 inhibitor.

How Supplied

Solifenacin is supplied as 5-mg and 10-mg tablets for oral use.

Prescribing Considerations

Solifenacin dose will have to be reduced for individuals with hepatic and renal impairment.

Because many medications are metabolized via CYP3A4, a careful medication history should be taken prior to beginning solifenacin.

Other medications are available for the treatment of OAB that may have a different dosing schedule and cost. Choice of medication should be individualized to the specific needs of each woman.

Cost: $$$$$

Spironolactone (Aldactone)

Therapeutic class: Antihypertensive

Chemical class: Potassium-sparing diuretic

Indications

Spironolactone is indicated for the management of:

1. Primary hyperaldosteronism
2. Edematous conditions associated with cirrhosis of the liver with edema/ascites, congestive heart failure (CHF), essential hypertension, hypokalemia, nephrotic syndrome, and severe heart failure.

Spironolactone has been used off label for the treatment of acne and hirsutism.

Contraindications

Spironolactone is contraindicated for individuals with acute renal insufficiency, anuria, hyperkalemia, or significant impairment of renal excretory function.

Mechanism of Action

Spironolactone acts through competitive binding of receptors at the aldosterone-dependent sodium-potassium exchange site in the renal tubule. It causes increased amounts of sodium and water to be excreted, while potassium is retained. Spironolactone acts as a diuretic and as an antihypertensive drug.

Spironolactone affects androgen receptors in the sebaceous glands, causing reduced sebum production and thereby improvement in acne symptoms. Spironolactone also blocks the development of more potent androgens in peripheral tissues, which may reduce hirsutism.

Metabolism & Excretion

Hepatic and renal

Adverse Reactions

Adverse reactions can include gynecomastia, hyperkalemia, hyponatremia, and hypotension.

Side Effects

Diarrhea, dizziness, nausea

Drug–Drug Interactions

Spironolactone is a potassium-sparing diuretic; therefore, potassium supplementation, either in the form of medication or as a diet rich in potassium, should not ordinarily occur with spironolactone.

Spironolactone should not be administered concurrently with other potassium-sparing diuretics.

Concomitant use with angiotensin converting enzyme (ACE) inhibitors or indomethacin increases the risk of severe hyperkalemia.

Spironolactone may increase the half-life of digoxin.

The concomitant use of nonsteroidal anti-inflammatory drugs (NSAIDs) and spironolactone may reduce the diuretic and antihypertensive effect of spironolactone.

Use of spironolactone with lithium may reduce the renal clearance of lithium and increase the risk of toxicity.

Use with central nervous system (CNS) agents may increase the risk of orthostatic hypotension.

The concurrent use of spironolactone and corticosteroids may increase electrolyte depletion and increase the risk of hypokalemia.

Specific Considerations for Women

Pregnancy

There are no adequate, well-controlled studies of spironolactone use by women who are pregnant. Spironolactone has endocrine effects in animals, including progestational and antiandrogenic effects, and could potentially cause feminization of a fetus who is male. Diuretics are generally not given during pregnancy and are not appropriate for the treatment of pregnancy-associated edema. Other antihypertensive agents, such as labetalol, can be considered for the management of chronic hypertension during pregnancy. Topical agents can be considered for the treatment of acne during pregnancy.

Breastfeeding

Spironolactone is excreted in breast milk in low amounts. Due to tumorigenic effects in animal studies, the product labeling advises against the use of spironolactone by women who are breastfeeding. If using spironolactone for the treatment of acne and hirsutism, consider the use of topical agents during lactation.

Adolescent women
Although product labeling states that safety and efficacy have not been established among the pediatric population, spironolactone has been used off label for the treatment of acne by adolescent women.

Elderly women
There are no differences in safety and efficacy among individuals who are older compared with individuals who are younger. However, individuals who are elderly may have more comorbid conditions that could increase the potential for adverse effects of spironolactone.

Dose: Variable, depending on condition being treated
Acne and hirsutism:
There is no established dose for acne or hirsutism because both indications are off label. In the literature, common doses of spironolactone for acne and hirsutism are 25 mg to 200 mg per day. Higher doses are often divided. Spironolactone 50 mg twice per day is a common dose that appears to provide a high rate of acne clearance and a low incidence of side effects.

Diagnosis of primary hyperaldosteronism:
Long test: 400 mg spironolactone is administered orally daily for 3 to 4 weeks. Correction of hypokalemia and of hypertension provides presumptive evidence for the diagnosis of primary hyperaldosteronism.

Short test: 400 mg spironolactone is administered orally daily for 4 days. If serum potassium increases during spironolactone administration but drops when spironolactone is discontinued, a presumptive diagnosis of primary hyperaldosteronism should be considered.

Edema related to heart failure, hepatic cirrhosis, and nephrotic syndrome:
The initial daily dose of spironolactone is 100 mg orally in either a single or divided dose. After 5 days, adjustments in dose can be made based on response. Typical range is 25 mg to 200 mg per day.

Essential hypertension:
The initial daily dose of spironolactone is 50 mg to 100 mg orally in either a single or divided dose.

Hypokalemia:
Doses of 25 mg to 100 mg daily are used for the treatment of diuretic-induced hypokalemia.

Severe heart failure:
Initial treatment includes 25 mg orally once daily if the serum potassium is less than or equal to 5.0 mEq/L and the serum creatinine is less than or equal to 2.5 mg/dL. If 25 mg once daily is tolerated, the dose may be increased to 50 mg once daily as clinically indicated.

How Supplied
Spironolactone is supplied as 25-mg, 50-mg, and 100-mg tablets for oral use.

Prescribing Considerations
Spironolactone has a **black box warning** for being tumorigenic in rat toxicity studies. The product labeling advises use only in approved conditions and avoidance of unnecessary use. How this observation in animals relates to use in humans is unknown.

The most common use of spironolactone among young women is in the off-label treatment of acne.

The use of spironolactone for the treatment of acne appears to be most effective in the setting of androgen sensitivity.

Individuals taking spironolactone should be cautioned to avoid large quantities of foods containing high amounts of potassium.

Cost: $

Sulfamethoxazole-trimethoprim (Bactrim, Bactrim DS)

Therapeutic class: Antibacterial

Chemical class: Sulfonamide

Indications
Sulfamethoxazole-trimethoprim (SMZ-TMP) is used to treat the following conditions caused by susceptible bacteria:

1. Urinary tract infections (UTIs)
2. Acute otitis media (AOM)
3. Acute exacerbations of chronic bronchitis among adults
4. Shigellosis
5. *Pneumocystis jiroveci* pneumonia
6. Traveler's diarrhea among adults

Contraindications
SMZ-TMP is contraindicated for individuals with a known allergy or hypersensitivity to sulfonamides or trimethoprim, for those with a history of drug-induced immune thrombocytopenia with use of sulfonamides and/or trimethoprim, and for individuals with documented megaloblastic anemia due to folate deficiency.

Sulfonamide antibiotics, including SMZ-TMP, should not be used for treatment of group A β-hemolytic streptococcal infections.

Mechanism of Action
Sulfamethoxazole inhibits bacterial synthesis of dihydrofolic acid, and trimethoprim blocks the production of tetrahydrofolic acid from dihydrofolic acid. Combined, SMZ-TMP blocks two consecutive steps in the biosynthesis of nucleic acids and proteins essential to many bacteria.

Metabolism & Excretion
Hepatic and renal

Adverse Reactions
Fatal hypersensitivity reactions have been reported with SMZ-TMP.

Clostridium difficile-associated diarrhea (CDAD) has been reported with the use of nearly all antibacterial agents, including SMZ-TMP.

Side Effects
Diarrhea, nausea, photosensitivity, skin rashes, and vomiting. Overgrowth of fungi can cause oral thrush and vulvovaginal candidiasis.

S

Drug–Drug Interactions

Co-administration of SMZ-TMP and leucovorin during treatment of *Pneumocystis jiroveci* pneumonia should be avoided.

Trimethoprim is an inhibitor of CYP2C8 as well as OCT2 transporter. Sulfamethoxazole is an inhibitor of CYP2C9. Interactions may occur when SMZ-TMP is co-administered with drugs that are substrates of CYP2C8 and 2C9 or OCT2.

Other drug interactions exist. The full prescribing information should be reviewed.

Specific Considerations for Women

Pregnancy

SMZ-TMP may interfere with folic acid metabolism. Some retrospective data have suggested an association between fetal SMZ-TMP exposure during the first trimester and an increased incidence of abnormalities, including club foot, neural tube defects, and oral clefts, although these effects have not been seen in other studies. Due to the conflicting data on potentially serious defects, SMZ-TMP should be avoided during pregnancy unless no other antibacterial agent is appropriate.

Breastfeeding

SMZ-TMP is excreted in breast milk and can be administered to infants beginning at 2 months of age. It should be avoided in the immediate neonatal period (first week after birth) due to the risk of hemolysis. SMZ-TMP use by women who are breastfeeding is acceptable with healthy, full-term infants after this time. SMZ-TMP should be avoided by women who are breastfeeding if the infant is ill, jaundiced, or premature. It should also be avoided if the infant has glucose-6-phosphate dehydrogenase (G6PD) deficiency.

Adolescent women

SMZ-TMP may be used by adolescent women.

Elderly women

No differences in safety or effectiveness have been noted between older and younger women. However, the risk of severe adverse reactions, such as blood disorders, electrolyte imbalances, and folic acid deficiency, may be more frequent among the elderly.

Dose

The dose is variable and based on the underlying infection being treated.

Generally, SMZ-TMP is given orally every 12 hours as either two SMZ-TMP tablets or one SMZ-TMP double-strength (DS) tablet. Length of treatment varies and is often between 5 to 14 days.

How Supplied

SMZ-TMP is supplied as a fixed-dose tablet for oral use containing 400 mg of sulfamethoxazole and 80 mg of trimethoprim.

SMZ-TMP DS is supplied as a fixed-dose tablet for oral use containing 800 mg of sulfamethoxazole and 160 mg of trimethoprim.

Prescribing Considerations

The full course of SMZ-TMP should be completed even if symptoms resolve prior to the end of treatment.

Fluids should be increased to prevent crystalluria and stone formation.

To avoid potentially serious hypersensitivity reactions, SMZ-TMP should be discontinued at the first sign of a skin rash.

Increased photosensitivity may occur, and exposure to natural and artificial sunlight should be avoided.

Cost: $

Sumatriptan (Imitrex)

Therapeutic class: Antimigraine

Chemical class: Serotonin (5-HT1B/1D) receptor agonist (triptan). Other medications in this category include almotriptan, eletriptan, naratriptan, and zolmitriptan.

Indications

Sumatriptan is indicated for the treatment of adult migraine, with or without aura.

Contraindications

Sumatriptan is contraindicated for individuals with:

1. Ischemic coronary artery disease (CAD) (angina pectoris, history of myocardial infarction, or documented silent ischemia) or coronary artery vasospasm
2. Wolff-Parkinson-White syndrome or arrhythmias associated with conduction pathway disorders
3. History of stroke or transient ischemic attack (TIA) or history of hemiplegic or basilar migraine because these individuals are at a higher risk of stroke
4. Peripheral vascular disease
5. Ischemic bowel disease
6. Uncontrolled hypertension
7. Recent (past 24 hours) use of ergotamine-containing medication, ergot-type medication, or another 5-hydroxytryptamine1 (5-HT1) agonist
8. Concurrent administration of a monoamine oxidase inhibitor (MAOI) or recent (within 2 weeks) use of an MAOI
9. Hypersensitivity or allergy to sumatriptan
10. Severe hepatic impairment

Mechanism of Action

Sumatriptan exerts therapeutic effects in the treatment of migraine headache through agonist effects at the 5-HT1B/1D receptors on intracranial blood vessels and sensory nerves of the trigeminal system. This results in cranial vessel constriction and inhibition of pro-inflammatory neuropeptide release.

Metabolism & Excretion

Hepatic and renal

Adverse Reactions

Serious adverse reactions can include anaphylaxis, cardiac arrhythmias, cerebrovascular events, chest tightness and pain, hypertension, increased headaches, myocardial infarction (MI), seizures, serotonin syndrome, and vasospasm reactions.

Side Effects

Pain in the throat, neck, or jaw; palpitations; paresthesias

Drug–Drug Interactions

MAOIs significantly increase systemic exposure of sumatriptan and should not be used concurrently.

Ergot-containing drugs and other 5-HT1 agonists (triptans) can prolong vasospastic reactions and should not be taken within 24 hours of sumatriptan.

Co-administration of triptans and MAOIs, selective serotonin reuptake inhibitors (SSRIs), serotonin norepinephrine reuptake inhibitors (SNRIs), or tricyclic antidepressants (TCAs) can increase the risk of serotonin syndrome.

Specific Considerations for Women

Pregnancy

Results of pregnancy registry data and meta-analysis of research results suggest that the use of triptans during pregnancy does not increase the risk of major birth defects or prematurity. With all medications during pregnancy, the lowest dose for the shortest time is always prudent.

Breastfeeding

Sumatriptan is present in breast milk in low levels after subcutaneous injection, but information is lacking about excretion in breast milk after oral doses. Sumatriptan has poor oral bioavailability. Intermittent use is not expected to cause adverse effects for an infant who is full term.

Adolescent women

Efficacy of sumatriptan for the treatment of migraine headache for individuals under 18 years of age has not been established.

Elderly women

There have been no observed differences in response to sumatriptan between younger and older individuals. Older individuals with preexisting cardiac risk factors (diabetes, hypertension, obesity, smoking) should be evaluated carefully prior to beginning treatment with sumatriptan.

Dose

Treatment can be initiated with either 25-mg, 50-mg, or 100-mg doses. If there is no headache relief after 2 hours, the dose can be repeated. Doses can be adjusted based on response and tolerance.

The maximum daily dose is 200 mg in a 24-hour period.

A maximum single dose should not exceed 50 mg in the presence of mild to moderate hepatic impairment.

How Supplied

Sumatriptan is supplied as 25-mg, 50-mg, and 100-mg tablets for oral use.

Prescribing Considerations

Sumatriptan is not indicated for the prevention of migraine headache.

If more than 4 migraine headaches occur within a 30-day period, additional and/or different treatment modalities should be considered.

Individuals who have multiple cardiac risk factors should be evaluated for cardiac disease prior to treatment. If there are multiple risks but no evidence of active cardiac disease, consider administering sumatriptan in a supervised clinical setting and obtaining an electrocardiogram (ECG) after the first dose.

Cost: $$

Tamoxifen (Nolvadex)

Therapeutic class: Antineoplastic

Chemical class: Estrogen agonist/antagonist; selective estrogen receptor modulator (SERM); other medications in this class include raloxifene.

Indications

Tamoxifen is indicated for adult women:

1. For treatment of estrogen receptor-positive metastatic breast cancer
2. For adjuvant treatment of early-stage estrogen receptor-positive breast cancer

3. To reduce risk of invasive breast cancer following breast surgery and radiation with ductal carcinoma in situ (DCIS)
4. To reduce the incidence of breast cancer if at high risk

Contraindications

Tamoxifen is contraindicated for women who require concomitant warfarin therapy or have a history of deep vein thrombosis (DVT) or pulmonary embolus (PE), if the indication for treatment is either reduction of breast cancer incidence for high-risk individuals or risk reduction of invasive breast cancer after treatment of DCIS.

Tamoxifen is also contraindicated with a known allergy or hypersensitivity to the medication.

Mechanism of Action

Tamoxifen competes with estrogen for binding to the estrogen receptor, which can result in a decrease in estrogen receptor signaling-dependent growth in breast tissue.

Metabolism & Excretion

Hepatic and gastrointestinal (fecal)

Adverse Reactions

The most serious potential adverse reactions include endometrial hyperplasia; elevated liver enzymes; hepatocellular carcinoma; hypercalcemia; leukopenia; ocular disturbances, including corneal changes; thrombocytopenia; thromboembolic events (DVT, PE, stroke); uterine carcinoma; and uterine polyps.

Side Effects

Bone pain, dizziness, hot flashes/flushes, menstrual cycle changes, nausea, vaginal dryness

Drug–Drug Interactions

Tamoxifen may reduce the plasma concentration of letrozole and increase the anticoagulant effect of warfarin.

Strong CYP3A4 inducers reduce the efficacy of tamoxifen and should not be used concurrently. The efficacy of tamoxifen may also be reduced with the co-administration of strong CYP2D6 inhibitors.

Specific Considerations for Women

Pregnancy

Tamoxifen can cause fetal harm and should not be used during pregnancy. Tamoxifen has been linked to spontaneous abortion, birth defects, and fetal death.

Breastfeeding

Tamoxifen has anti-estrogen properties and may suppress lactation. It should not be used by women who are breastfeeding.

Adolescent women

Conditions for which tamoxifen is used do not generally occur during adolescence. Safety and efficacy have not been established for women under age 18.

Elderly women

No differences in efficacy or tolerability have been established between women under age 65 and women over age 65.

Dose

The dose for adjuvant treatment of breast cancer, DCIS, and reduction of breast cancer incidence for women at high risk is 20 mg orally daily.

The dose for treatment of metastatic breast cancer is 20 mg to 40 mg orally daily. Doses greater than 20 mg per day should be administered in divided doses (morning and evening).

How Supplied

Tamoxifen is available in 10-mg and 20-mg tablets for oral use.

Prescribing Considerations

Tamoxifen has a **black box warning** for the risk of endometrial adenocarcinoma, PE, stroke, and uterine sarcoma. For most women who have received a definitive diagnosis of breast cancer, the benefits of tamoxifen outweigh the risks. Women who do not have breast cancer but are considering the use of tamoxifen for risk reduction should weigh the risks versus possible benefits.

Length of treatment is 5 years for most indications.

Women of reproductive potential need to use effective nonhormonal contraception during treatment with tamoxifen and for 9 months following the last dose. A negative pregnancy test should be documented prior to beginning treatment with tamoxifen.

Tamoxifen does not eliminate the risk of breast cancer. Women should have a clinical breast exam and mammogram prior to starting tamoxifen and continue with regular breast exams and mammograms during treatment per national guidelines.

Abnormal uterine bleeding should be reported to a healthcare provider and investigated appropriately.

Annual gynecologic exams are prudent.

Cost: $$

Terconazole (Terazol)

Therapeutic class: Antifungal

Chemical class: Azole antifungal

Indications
Terconazole is indicated for the local treatment of vulvovaginal candidiasis.

Contraindications
Terconazole is contraindicated for women who are known to be hypersensitive to terconazole or to any component of the cream or suppositories.

Mechanism of Action
Terconazole inhibits the fungal cytochrome P-450-mediated by the 14 alpha-lanosterol demethylase enzyme. The inhibition of this enzyme results in the loss of ergosterol in the fungal cell wall and may be responsible for the antifungal activity of terconazole.

T

Metabolism & Excretion
Hepatic and renal/gastrointestinal (fecal)

Adverse Reactions
Rare cases of anaphylaxis and toxic epidermal necrolysis have been reported during terconazole therapy.

Side Effects
The most common side effects are vulvovaginal burning, irritation, and itching, which are the most frequent reasons for discontinuation of treatment.

Drug–Drug Interactions
There are no known drug–drug interactions with terconazole.

Specific Considerations for Women
Pregnancy
No teratogenicity has been noted in animal studies. According to package labeling, terconazole should be used only in the second or third trimester of pregnancy, although azole antifungal medications are generally considered safe during pregnancy.

Breastfeeding
It is not known if terconazole is excreted in breast milk. Limited systemic absorption from short-term vaginal preparations is expected. However, another azole, such as miconazole, has poor oral bioavailability and is unlikely to adversely affect an infant who is breastfeeding.

Adolescent women
Terconazole may be used by adolescent women.

Elderly women
No differences in safety or effectiveness have been noted between older and younger women.

Dose
Each preparation is used intravaginally at bedtime for 3 to 7 consecutive nights depending on formulation.

How Supplied

Terconazole is available as:

7-day vaginal cream 0.4%

3-day vaginal cream 0.8%

3 vaginal suppositories 80 mg each

Prescribing Considerations

The suppository formulation (not the cream) may damage diaphragms or latex condoms and should not be used concurrently with those forms of contraception.

Terconazole can be used during menstruation, but tampons should be avoided because they absorb the medication and may reduce efficacy.

Cost: $

Tinidazole (Tindamax)

Therapeutic class: Antiprotozoal

Chemical class: Nitroimidazole; other medications in this category include metronidazole and secnidazole.

Indications

Tinidazole is indicated for the treatment of amebiasis, bacterial vaginosis (BV), giardiasis, and trichomoniasis.

Contraindications

Tinidazole is contraindicated for individuals with a previous history of hypersensitivity to tinidazole or other nitroimidazole derivatives.

Tinidazole is contraindicated during the first trimester of pregnancy, and safer alternatives should be considered for the remainder of the pregnancy. Tinidazole should not be used by women who are breastfeeding.

Mechanism of Action

Tinidazole has antiprotozoal and antibacterial properties. The nitro-group of tinidazole is reduced by cell extracts of trichomonas, which may be

T

responsible for the antiprotozoal activity. Chemically reduced tinidazole releases nitrites and causes damage to bacterial DNA in vitro. Additionally, the drug causes DNA base changes in bacterial cells and DNA strand breakage.

Metabolism & Excretion
Hepatic and renal

Adverse Reactions
Convulsive seizures and peripheral neuropathy have been reported by individuals treated with tinidazole.

Tinidazole may produce transient leukopenia and neutropenia and should be used with caution by individuals with current or a history of blood dyscrasias.

Side Effects
The use of tinidazole may result in vulvovaginal candidiasis. Gastrointestinal (GI) side effects include abdominal pain, diarrhea, metallic or bitter taste, nausea, and vomiting. Dizziness, fatigue, headaches, and malaise have been reported.

Drug–Drug Interactions
The following drug interactions were reported for metronidazole, a chemically related nitroimidazole. It is possible these drug interactions may occur with tinidazole:

Alcohol may cause a disulfiram-like reaction and should be avoided during treatment and for 3 days after completion of the medication.

Metronidazole has been reported to potentiate the anticoagulant effect of warfarin and other oral coumarin anticoagulants, which can result in prolongation of prothrombin time.

Metronidazole may increase the serum concentration of busulfan and lithium.

Drugs that inhibit CYP450 enzymes, such as cimetidine, may prolong the half-life and decrease plasma clearance of metronidazole.

Drugs that induce CYP450 enzymes, such as phenobarbital or phenytoin, may increase the elimination of metronidazole and reduce plasma levels.

Specific Considerations for Women
Pregnancy
Data from studies involving human subjects are limited regarding use of tinidazole during pregnancy; however, animal data suggest that this drug poses moderate risk. Thus, tinidazole should be avoided during the first trimester by women who are pregnant. The use of tinidazole in the second and third trimesters of pregnancy should be weighed against the possible risks to both the mother and the fetus. Consider other options that have a more favorable safety profile, such as metronidazole, for treatment of BV or trichomoniasis.

Breastfeeding
Amounts of tinidazole in breast milk are less than doses given to infants. No research has evaluated the effects of tinidazole for infants who are breastfeeding. However, the closely related drug metronidazole causes an increased risk of oral *Candida* infections. Additionally, concern has been raised about exposure of infants who are healthy to tinidazole in breast milk because of possible mutagenicity and carcinogenicity. Breastfeeding should be deferred for 72 hours following a single 2-gram dose of tinidazole and for 3 days after the last dose in a multi-day regimen.

Adolescent women
Tinidazole can be used by adolescent women.

Elderly women
No differences in safety or effectiveness have been noted between older and younger women.

Dose: Variable, depending on condition being treated
Amebiasis (intestinal):
2 grams orally per day for 3 days with food

Amebic liver abscess:
2 grams orally per day for 3 to 5 days with food

Bacterial vaginosis:
2 grams once daily for 2 days taken with food, or 1 gram once daily for 5 days taken with food

Giardiasis:
A 2-gram single dose taken orally with food

Trichomoniasis:
A 2-gram single dose taken orally with food. Sexual partners also need treatment.

How Supplied
Tinidazole is supplied as 250-mg and 500-mg tablets for oral use.

Prescribing Considerations
Tinidazole has a **black box warning** because metronidazole, another nitro-imidazole agent, has been shown to be carcinogenic in mice and rats. Although carcinogenicity has not been reported for tinidazole, the two drugs are structurally related and have similar biologic effects. Per package labeling, unnecessary use of the drug should be avoided. How carcinogenicity in rats and mice relates to intermittent use of nitroimidazoles for humans is unknown.

Completing the full course of tinidazole is necessary.

Partners of women diagnosed with trichomoniasis must also be treated to prevent reinfection.

Inform women about the possible interaction with alcohol.

Taking tinidazole with food may decrease GI side effects.

Other nitroimidazole medications, such as metronidazole, are available that may have a different dosing schedule and cost. Choice of medication should be individualized to the specific needs of each woman.

Cost: $$

Topiramate (Topamax)

Therapeutic class: Antiepileptic

Chemical class: Sulfamate

Indications
Topiramate is indicated for:

1. Initial epilepsy monotherapy for individuals 2 years of age or older with partial-onset or primary generalized tonic-clonic seizures
2. Adjunctive epilepsy therapy for adults and children (2 to 16 years of age) with partial-onset seizures or primary generalized tonic-clonic seizures, and for individuals 2 years of age or older with seizures associated with Lennox-Gastaut syndrome (LGS)
3. Treatment for adults for prophylaxis of migraine headache

Contraindications
There are no known contraindications to use of topiramate.

Mechanism of Action
Topiramate blocks voltage-dependent sodium channels; augments the activity of the neurotransmitter gamma-aminobutyrate at subtypes of the GABA-A receptor; antagonizes the glutamate receptor; and inhibits the carbonic anhydrase enzyme, particularly isozymes II and IV.

Metabolism & Excretion
Not extensively metabolized and primarily excreted unchanged in the urine

Adverse Reactions
Potentially serious adverse reactions include acute myopia, hyperthermia, metabolic acidosis, neuropsychiatric symptoms (confusion, depression, fatigue, and somnolence), oligohidrosis, paresthesia, renal stones, secondary angle-closure glaucoma, sudden unexplained death, and suicidal behavior and ideation.

Side Effects
Abnormal taste, anorexia, dizziness, nervousness, weight loss

Drug–Drug Interactions
Decreased efficacy of combined hormonal contraception (CHC) and an increase in breakthrough bleeding can occur, especially at doses higher than 200 mg of topiramate per day.

Concomitant use of topiramate and valproic acid may cause hyperammonemia and hypothermia.

Concomitant administration of carbamazepine or phenytoin may decrease topiramate levels.

Alcohol and other central nervous system (CNS) depressants can potentiate the adverse neuropsychiatric and CNS effects of topiramate.

Concomitant use of topiramate, a carbonic anhydrase inhibitor, with any other carbonic anhydrase inhibitor may increase the severity of metabolic acidosis and may also increase the risk of renal stone formation.

Specific Considerations for Women
Pregnancy
Topiramate may cause fetal harm. Information from pregnancy registries suggests that topiramate is associated with fetal oral clefts. Topiramate should not be used for migraine prophylaxis during pregnancy. If topiramate is necessary for the control and treatment of epilepsy, women should be aware of the increased risk of fetal harm.

Breastfeeding
Doses up to 200 mg per day produce low levels of topiramate in breast milk. Lower doses have a lesser effect on breast milk. Diarrhea, inadequate weight gain, and irritability are possible for the infant who is breastfeeding. If using topiramate for migraine prophylaxis, consider the frequency of migraine headaches and the possibility of treating migraines with a different medication as they occur. Intermittent sumatriptan may be an alternative.

Adolescent women
Topiramate is not approved for migraine prophylaxis for adolescents. It is approved for the treatment of epilepsy for adolescents.

Elderly women
There is no evidence of differences in safety and efficacy between older and younger individuals. Elderly individuals with decreased renal function may need a dose reduction.

Dose

Adult epilepsy monotherapy:

The recommended dose is 400 mg orally daily in 2 divided doses. Titration schedule:

 Week 1: 25 mg orally in the morning and 25 mg in the evening
 Week 2: 50 mg orally in the morning and 50 mg in the evening
 Week 3: 75 mg orally in the morning and 75 mg in the evening
 Week 4: 100 mg orally in the morning and 100 mg in the evening
 Week 5: 150 mg orally in the morning and 150 mg in the evening
 Week 6: 200 mg orally in the morning and 200 mg in the evening

Adult (age 17 and older) epilepsy adjunct therapy:

The recommended dose for individuals with partial-onset seizures is 200 mg to 400 mg orally daily in 2 divided doses and 400 mg orally daily in 2 divided doses for primary generalized tonic-clonic seizures.

 Initial doses should begin at 25 mg to 50 mg orally daily and titrated to an effective dose in increments of 25 mg to 50 mg daily each week.

Migraine prophylaxis:

The recommended dose is 100 mg orally daily in 2 divided doses. Titration schedule:

 Week 1: 25 mg orally in the evening
 Week 2: 25 mg orally in the morning and 25 mg in the evening
 Week 3: 25 mg orally in the morning and 50 mg in the evening
 Week 4: 50 mg orally in the morning and 50 mg in the evening

 For individuals with renal impairment (creatinine clearance less than 70 ml/min/1.73 m^2), half of the usual adult dose is recommended.

How Supplied

Topiramate is supplied as 25-mg, 50-mg, 100-mg, and 200-mg tablets for oral use and sprinkle capsules in doses of 15 mg and 25 mg.

Prescribing Considerations

Topiramate should be discontinued gradually to reduce the risk of seizures that can occur with rapid withdrawal.

Women of reproductive potential who are sexually active should use an effective method of contraception while taking topiramate due to the increased risks of birth defects.

Topiramate may decrease the effectiveness of CHC and increase the risk of breakthrough bleeding. Contraceptive options should be reviewed.

If a woman becomes pregnant while taking topiramate, she should consider enrolling in the North American Antiepileptic Pregnancy Registry found at http://www.aedpregnancyregistry.org/.

Cost: $–$$

Tramadol (Ultram, Ultram ER)

Therapeutic class: Analgesic

Chemical class: Opioid

Indications
Tramadol is indicated for the treatment of adults with moderate to moderately severe pain.

Contraindications
Tramadol is contraindicated with a known hypersensitivity reaction to the medication or other opioids. It is also contraindicated in situations where opioids are contraindicated, including acute intoxication from alcohol, hypnotics, opioids, psychotropics, and/or sedatives.

Carbamazepine increases tramadol metabolism and seizure risk. Concomitant administration of tramadol and carbamazepine is not recommended.

Mechanism of Action
Tramadol exerts an analgesic effect through binding μ-opioid receptors and weak inhibition of reuptake of norepinephrine and serotonin.

Metabolism & Excretion
Hepatic and renal

Adverse Reactions
Potentially serious adverse reactions include anaphylaxis, respiratory depression, seizures, and serotonin syndrome.

Side Effects
Constipation, dizziness, drowsiness, dry mouth, headache, nausea, somnolence, vomiting

Drug–Drug Interactions
Seizure risk is increased when tramadol is taken concomitantly with monoamine oxidase inhibitors (MAOIs), neuroleptics, other opioids, selective serotonin reuptake inhibitors (SSRIs), and tricyclic antidepressants (TCAs) and other tricyclic compounds.

Use with central nervous system (CNS) depressants, including alcohol, other opioids, phenothiazines, sedative hypnotics, or tranquilizers, increases the risk of CNS depression.

Concomitant administration of CYP2D6 and/or CYP3A4 inhibitors, such as amitriptyline, fluoxetine, paroxetine, and quinidine (CYP2D6 inhibitors), and erythromycin and ketoconazole (CYP3A4 inhibitors), may reduce metabolic clearance of tramadol and increase the risk for serious adverse events, including seizures and serotonin syndrome.

Specific Considerations for Women
Pregnancy
There are no adequate, well-controlled studies of tramadol use by women who are pregnant. Fetal death, neonatal seizures, neonatal withdrawal syndrome, and stillbirth have been reported during postmarketing. Therefore, tramadol should be used during pregnancy only if the potential benefit justifies the potential risk to the fetus.

Breastfeeding
Tramadol is excreted in breast milk in low levels. Although these levels are unlikely to cause any adverse effects for the infant, the Food and Drug Administration (FDA) has advised women against breastfeeding while taking tramadol.

Adolescent women
Tramadol is approved for use by individuals age 17 and older.

Elderly women
Individuals over 75 years of age exhibit elevated serum concentrations and a prolonged elimination half-life of tramadol. Reductions in the daily dose are recommended for individuals older than 75 years.

Dose
Suggested dosing immediate release:
Initiate tramadol at 25 mg orally per day in the morning and titrate in 25-mg increments in separate doses every 3 days to reach 100 mg per day (25 mg four times per day). Thereafter, the total daily dose may be increased by 50 mg as tolerated every 3 days to reach 200 mg per day (50 mg four times per day). After titration, tramadol in doses of 50 mg to 100 mg can be administered as needed for pain relief every 4 to 6 hours. Total daily dose should not exceed 400 mg per day.

Suggested dosing extended release:
Initiate tramadol ER at a dose of 100 mg orally once daily and titrate up as necessary by 100-mg increments every 5 days depending upon tolerability and pain relief. Total daily dose should not exceed 300 mg per day.

Individuals with creatinine clearances of less than 30 ml/min should not exceed 200 mg per day.

Individuals who are older, especially those over 75 years of age, should not exceed 300 mg per day.

How Supplied
Tramadol is supplied as an immediate-release 50-mg tablet for oral use.

Tramadol ER is supplied as 100-mg, 200-mg, and 300-mg extended-release tablets for oral use.

Prescribing Considerations
Women appear to have a higher peak tramadol concentration compared to men. Consider whether a lower dose may be prudent for women.

Tramadol may impair cognitive and physical functions. Activities that require mental alertness should be avoided until it is known how tramadol affects these functions.

Tramadol has mu-opioid agonist activity and the potential for abuse.

Tramadol should be tapered to avoid withdrawal symptoms (abdominal cramps, diarrhea, nausea, pain, sweating) that can occur with abrupt discontinuation.

Administration of naloxone for tramadol overdose will reverse some symptoms but may also increase the risk for seizures.

Cost: $$

Tranexamic acid (Lysteda)

Therapeutic class: Hemostatic

Chemical class: Antifibrinolytic

Indications
Tranexamic acid is indicated for the treatment of cyclic, heavy menstrual bleeding (HMB).

Contraindications
Tranexamic acid increases clotting. Therefore, tranexamic acid is contraindicated for women:

1. Taking combined hormonal contraception (CHC)
2. With active thromboembolic disease, a history of thromboembolism, or intrinsic risk of thromboembolism (hypercoagulopathy, thrombotic valvular or cardiac disease)

Risk of thrombosis may also be increased for women taking Factor IX complex concentrates, anti-inhibitor coagulant concentrates, and all-trans retinoic acid for acute promyelocytic leukemia.

T

Mechanism of Action
Tranexamic acid is a synthetic lysine amino acid derivative. The medication results in the occupation of lysine receptor binding sites of plasmin for fibrin. This leads to stabilization and preservation of fibrin in blood clots, which helps reduce bleeding.

Metabolism & Excretion
Hepatic (limited) and renal

Adverse Reactions
Thromboembolic events have occurred, including retinal artery and retinal vein occlusions and arterial and venous thromboembolism.

Side Effects
Abdominal pain, back pain, generalized musculoskeletal pain, headache, nasal and sinus congestion

Drug–Drug Interactions
In addition to CHCs, Factor IX complex concentrates, anti-inhibitor co-agulant concentrates, and all-trans retinoic acid for acute promyelocytic leukemia discussed previously, concomitant therapy with tissue plasminogen activators may decrease the efficacy of tranexamic acid and the tissue plasminogen activators.

Specific Considerations for Women
Pregnancy
Tranexamic acid is not indicated during pregnancy because women who are pregnant do not have a menstrual cycle. However, there is no indication of fetal harm if tranexamic acid is taken during early pregnancy.

Breastfeeding
Tranexamic acid is present in breast milk in very small amounts. No adverse outcomes have been documented for infants who are breastfeeding. Women who require tranexamic acid to control HMB do not need to discontinue breastfeeding or discard milk.

Adolescent women
No dose adjustments are needed for adolescent women.

Elderly women

Tranexamic acid is not indicated for use by women who are postmenopausal because they do not have a menstrual cycle.

Dose

The dose for women with normal renal function is 1,300 mg (two 650-mg tablets) three times a day (total of 3,900 mg per day) for a maximum of 5 days during menstruation.

In the presence of renal impairment, the dose is based on serum creatinine and adjusted as follows:

Creatinine above 1.4 mg/dL and less than or equal to 2.8 mg/dL: 1,300 mg (two 650-mg tablets) two times a day (2,600 per day) for a maximum of 5 days during menstruation.

Creatinine above 2.8 mg/dL and less than or equal to 5.7 mg/dL: 1,300 mg (two 650-mg tablets) once a day (1,300 mg per day) for a maximum of 5 days during menstruation.

Creatinine above 5.7 mg/dL: 650 mg (one 650-mg tablet) once a day (650 mg per day) for a maximum of 5 days during menstruation.

How Supplied

Tranexamic acid is available as 650-mg tablets for oral use.

Prescribing Considerations

Endometrial pathology as a cause of HMB should be excluded prior to beginning treatment with tranexamic acid.

Estrogen-containing contraception is contraindicated for women taking tranexamic acid. Other forms of contraception that do not contain estrogen should be discussed.

Cost: $$

Tretinoin (Renova, Retin-A Cream, Gel)

Therapeutic class: Anti-acne

Chemical class: Retinoid

Indications

Tretinoin cream (0.025%, 0.05%, and 0.1%) and gel (0.01% and 0.025%) are indicated for topical application in the treatment of acne vulgaris.

Tretinoin cream 0.02% is indicated as an adjunctive agent for use in the mitigation of fine facial wrinkles for individuals who use comprehensive skin care and avoid solar damage.

Contraindications

Tretinoin is contraindicated with a known allergy or hypersensitivity to the medication.

Mechanism of Action

Topical tretinoin decreases cohesiveness of follicular epithelial cells, which decreases comedone formation. Additionally, tretinoin stimulates increased turnover of follicular epithelial cells, causing extrusion of the comedones.

Topical tretinoin is also involved in keratin inhibition, which helps reduce fine lines and hyperpigmentation.

Metabolism & Excretion

Minimally excreted in urine

Adverse Reactions

No serious adverse reactions have been noted.

Side Effects

Skin reactions are common and can include blistering, crusting, dryness, edema, pigment changes, and redness. Heightened susceptibility to sunlight is common.

Drug–Drug Interactions

Concomitant use of tretinoin with other topical medications, medicated or abrasive soaps/cleaners, and cosmetics that have a strong drying effect should be avoided, as should products with high concentrations of alcohol, astringents, salicylic acid, and sulfur.

Use with other medications that increase skin photosensitivity, such as fluoroquinolones, sulfonamides, and tetracyclines, should be avoided.

Specific Considerations for Women
Pregnancy
Topical tretinoin has been associated with fetal abnormalities in animal models, and the observational data from humans are inconclusive. Acne treatment is not a necessity during pregnancy and topical tretinoin should be avoided. Other topical agents with a known safety profile, such as benzoyl peroxide or erythromycin, can be considered for acne treatment.

Breastfeeding
Tretinoin is poorly absorbed after topical application, and topical use has a low risk of causing adverse effects for the infant who is breastfeeding.

Adolescent women
Topical application of tretinoin for the treatment of acne is acceptable for adolescent women.

Elderly women
Women who are older may use topical tretinoin to reduce fine wrinkles and hyperpigmentation. Older skin may be more susceptible to damage and the drying effects of tretinoin.

Dose
Tretinoin is applied in a thin layer to the affected area each night at bedtime.

How Supplied
Tretinoin cream is available in 0.025%, 0.05%, and 0.1% strengths in 20-gram and 45-gram tubes.

Tretinoin cream 0.02% is available in 20-gram, 40-gram, and 60-gram tubes and a 44-gram pump.

Tretinoin gel is available in 0.01% and 0.025% strengths in 20-gram and 45-gram tubes.

Prescribing Considerations
There is an increased risk of sunburn when exposed to natural or artificial sunlight. Sun exposure should be limited, and skin should be protected with clothing and sunscreen.

Treatment with tretinoin may make skin more sensitive to wind and cold temperatures.

Frequent washing of the affected area with harsh products should be avoided.

If excessive dryness or irritation occurs, tretinoin can be applied every other night.

Tretinoin 0.02% cream will not remove wrinkles completely or repair sun-damaged skin. It could take up to 6 months to see results, and any improvement will disappear when treatment is stopped.

Cost: $$$

Ulipristal acetate (Ella)

Therapeutic class: Emergency contraceptive

Chemical class: Progesterone agonist/antagonist

Indications
Ulipristal acetate is an emergency contraceptive indicated for the prevention of pregnancy after unprotected intercourse or a known or suspected contraceptive failure.

Contraindications
Ulipristal acetate should not be used with a known or suspected pregnancy because its purpose is the prevention of pregnancy. It is not indicated for the termination of pregnancy.

Mechanism of Action
The primary mechanism of action of ulipristal acetate for emergency contraception is the probable inhibition or delay of ovulation. When ulipristal acetate is taken prior to ovulation, it delays follicular rupture. Implantation may also be affected due to alterations to the endometrium.

Metabolism & Excretion
Hepatic and gastrointestinal (fecal)

Adverse Reactions
No serious adverse reactions have been reported with ulipristal acetate when used for emergency contraception.

Side Effects
The most common side effects include abdominal pain, dysmenorrhea, headache, and nausea.

Drug–Drug Interactions
Ulipristal acetate is predominantly metabolized by CYP3A4. Therefore, drugs and supplements that are CYP3A4 inducers may decrease plasma concentration of ulipristal acetate and decrease effectiveness. These include barbiturates, bosentan, carbamazepine, felbamate, griseofulvin, oxcarbazepine, phenytoin, rifampin, St. John's wort, and topiramate.

Medications that are CYP3A4 inhibitors, including itraconazole and ketoconazole, can increase plasma concentrations of ulipristal acetate.

Specific Considerations for Women
Pregnancy
There is no conclusive evidence that ulipristal acetate results in congenital anomalies or pregnancy failure if taken after pregnancy has been established. It is not indicated for the termination of pregnancy.

Breastfeeding
Ulipristal acetate is excreted in breast milk. Women who are breastfeeding and take ulipristal acetate should pump and discard the milk for 24 hours after taking the medication.

Adolescent women
Ulipristal acetate can be used by adolescent women.

Elderly women
Ulipristal acetate can be used by perimenopausal women who are at risk for an unintended pregnancy. It is not indicated for postmenopausal women who are not at risk for pregnancy.

U

Dose
The dose is one tablet taken orally as soon as possible, within 120 hours or 5 days after unprotected intercourse or contraceptive failure.

How Supplied
Ulipristal acetate is available as a 30-mg tablet for oral administration.

Prescribing Considerations
Ulipristal acetate and the progestin component of hormonal contraceptives both bind to progestin receptors, and using them concurrently could decreased the effectiveness of progestin-containing contraception and/or the ability of ulipristal acetate to prevent ovulation. Progestin-containing hormonal contraception should not be resumed or started for at least 1 day (or up to 5 days) after the administration of ulipristal acetate. A barrier method is indicated until hormonal contraception has been used for a full 7 days.

Fertility can return rapidly after taking ulipristal acetate, and women should not rely on this as a routine method of contraception.

Ulipristal acetate may be taken more than once in a menstrual cycle without evidence of harm, although its ability to prevent pregnancy may be diminished.

The efficacy of taking ulipristal acetate more than 120 hours (5 days) after unprotected intercourse isn't known exactly but is expected to be diminished.

Menses may be altered, either decreasing or increasing the length of the menstrual cycle by a few days. A pregnancy test should be done if menses don't occur within 3 weeks of taking ulipristal acetate.

Ulipristal acetate provides no protection against sexually transmitted infections (STIs) and HIV. If vomiting occurs within 2 hours of taking ulipristal acetate, women should speak with their healthcare provider about whether a repeated dose is warranted.

Ulipristal acetate may have limited availability in certain geographical areas. Women can access https://www.ellanow.com/ for information on how to obtain the medication if it is not available in a local pharmacy.

Valacyclovir (Valtrex)

Therapeutic class: Antiviral

Chemical class: Purine nucleotide analogue; other drugs in this category include acyclovir and famciclovir.

Indications
Valacyclovir is indicated for the treatment of:

1. Cold sores (herpes labialis)
2. Genital herpes (HSV), initial or recurrent episodes
3. HSV suppression in immunocompetent or individuals who are HIV-positive
4. Reduction of transmission of HSV
5. Herpes zoster (shingles)
6. Varicella (chicken pox)

Contraindications
Valacyclovir is contraindicated with a known allergy, anaphylactic reaction, or hypersensitivity to either the medication or acyclovir.

Mechanism of Action
Valacyclovir is rapidly converted to acyclovir, which inhibits DNA synthesis. Acyclovir stops replication of herpes viral DNA by inhibition of viral DNA polymerase, termination of the growing viral DNA chain, and inactivation of the viral DNA polymerase.

Metabolism & Excretion
Hepatic and renal

Adverse Reactions
Serious adverse reactions are possible.

Thrombotic thrombocytopenic purpura/hemolytic uremic syndrome (TTP/HUS) has been reported by individuals with advanced HIV, allogeneic

V

bone marrow transplant, and renal transplant recipients. Rarely, these reactions have been fatal.

Acute renal failure has been reported by individuals who are elderly, by those with renal disease receiving a dose that is too high, by individuals taking other nephrotoxic drugs, and by those without adequate hydration.

Central nervous system (CNS) reactions, including agitation, confusion, delirium, hallucinations, and seizures, have been reported by the elderly and by individuals with renal disease.

Side Effects
Abdominal pain, headache, nausea

Drug–Drug Interactions
There are no known clinically significant drug–drug interactions.

Specific Considerations for Women
Pregnancy
Valacyclovir can be used during pregnancy. Based on pregnancy registry data, valacyclovir does not appear to increase the rate of birth defects beyond what occurs in the general population. According to the American College of Obstetricians and Gynecologists (ACOG), women experiencing an initial HSV outbreak or recurrent HSV during pregnancy should be offered antiviral medication to decrease the risk of perinatal transmission.

Breastfeeding
According to the package labeling, valacyclovir should be administered with caution for a woman who is breastfeeding and used only when indicated. Systemic maternal acyclovir (converted from valacyclovir) is generally compatible with breastfeeding. Valacyclovir is used for conditions that affect the pediatric population. Neonates and infants who are breastfeeding can expect to receive less than 1% of the exposure obtained after administering an intravenous dose for the treatment of neonatal herpes.

Adolescent women
Valacyclovir can be used by adolescent women.

Elderly women
There are no reported differences in safety and efficacy between older and younger individuals. Individuals who are elderly (over age 65) are more likely to have reduced renal function than younger individuals and require dose reduction. Adverse CNS and renal events are more likely to occur among the elderly.

Dose: Variable, depending on condition being treated
Cold sores:
2 grams orally every 12 hours for one day

Genital HSV initial episode:
1 gram orally twice daily for 10 days

Genital HSV recurrent episodes:
500 mg orally twice daily for 3 days

Genital HSV suppression:
1 gram once daily or 500 mg orally once daily (up to 9 recurrences/year)

Genital HSV suppression in individuals who are HIV-positive:
500 mg orally once daily

Herpes zoster:
1 gram orally three times daily for 7 days

Varicella:
1 gram orally three times daily for 5 to 7 days

How Supplied
Valacyclovir is supplied as 500-mg and 1-gram caplets for oral administration.

Prescribing Considerations
Dose adjustments are required for individuals with decreased renal function. Valacyclovir prescribing information contains dose adjustments based on creatinine clearance.

V

Varicella infections tend to be more severe for adolescents and adults. For best response, initiate treatment with valacyclovir within 24 hours of disease onset.

Treatment for herpes zoster (shingles) should be initiated within 72 hours of disease onset.

Genital HSV outbreaks change in frequency and severity over time. Re-evaluate the woman after 1 year of suppressive therapy to determine the need for continuation of treatment.

Episodic treatment for HSV should begin at the earliest sign (prodrome) of an outbreak.

Other antiviral medications exist, such as acyclovir, which has a more frequent dosing schedule but may be less expensive. Choice of medication should be individualized to the specific needs of each woman.

Varenicline (Chantix)

Therapeutic class: Smoking cessation agent

Chemical class: Partial nicotinic acetylcholine receptor agonist

Indications
Varenicline is indicated as an aid in smoking cessation treatment.

Contraindications
History of hypersensitivity or skin reactions to the medication

Mechanism of Action
Varenicline prevents nicotine binding to nicotinic acetylcholine receptors. This blocks the ability of nicotine to stimulate the dopamine system and reward experienced with smoking.

Metabolism & Excretion
Metabolism is minimal; more than 90% of varenicline is excreted unchanged in urine.

Adverse Reactions

Serious adverse reactions have occurred, including neuropsychiatric symptoms of agitation, depression, hallucinations, hostility, mania, psychosis, and suicidal ideation. Individuals with a history of mental health disorders may experience increased adverse reactions.

Seizures have been reported, most occurring within the first month of treatment.

Angioedema and serious skin reactions have occurred.

Somnambulism, loss of consciousness, and accidental injury may occur.

Varenicline may increase cardiovascular risk for individuals with underlying cardiac disease.

Side Effects

Abdominal pain, difficulty concentrating, dizziness, dry mouth, flatulence, insomnia, nausea

Drug–Drug Interactions

Increased intoxicating effects may occur when used with alcohol. Otherwise, there are no known clinically significant drug–drug interactions.

Specific Considerations for Women

Pregnancy

Available data do not suggest an increased risk for major birth defects for infants whose mothers took varenicline during pregnancy, compared with women who smoke. Smoking during pregnancy increases the risk of fetal growth restriction, low birth weight, neonatal death, orofacial clefts, placenta previa, placental abruption, premature rupture of membranes, preterm delivery, stillbirth, and sudden infant death syndrome. It is not known whether using varenicline to assist with quitting smoking during pregnancy reduces these risks.

Breastfeeding

There are no data on the presence of varenicline in human milk, the effects on an infant who is breastfeeding, or the effects on milk quantity or quality. Other smoking cessation modalities should be considered prior to using varenicline while breastfeeding. Bupropion may be an alternative.

V

Adolescent women
Women age 16 and older may use varenicline. Adolescent women who are younger should consider other available options, including nicotine replacement.

Elderly women
No dose adjustments are recommended for women over age 65 and no differences in safety or effectiveness have been noted between older and younger women.

Dose
Varenicline should be initiated one week prior to chosen quit date. Usual dosing is as follows:
   Days 1–3: 0.5 mg orally once daily
   Days 4–7: 0.5 mg orally twice daily
   Day 8 to end of treatment: 1 mg orally twice daily

How Supplied
Varenicline is available in 0.5-mg and 1-mg tablets for oral use.

Prescribing Considerations
Women should be evaluated after an initial 12 weeks of treatment. If they have been successful in complete tobacco cessation, treatment is advised for an additional 12 weeks to increase the likelihood of long-term smoking cessation.

If women are unable to quit smoking completely with treatment, smoking should be gradually reduced over the course of 12 weeks while treatment continues.

Smokers who relapse after quitting may repeat treatment with varenicline.

Alcohol consumption should be avoided or reduced during treatment.

To reduce the risk for accidental injury, women should be counseled to avoid driving, operating machinery, or engaging in activities that require complete mental alertness until they know how varenicline will affect them.

If neuropsychiatric symptoms develop during treatment, varenicline should be stopped and the woman should be evaluated by a healthcare provider.